COLOUR ATLAS OF
WOUNDS AND WOUNDING

COLOUR ATLAS OF WOUNDS AND WOUNDING

G. Austin Gresham, TD, ScD, MD, FRCPath.

Professor of Morbid Anatomy and Histology
University of Cambridge

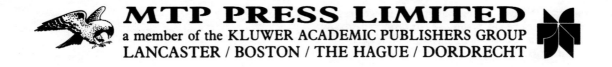

MTP PRESS LIMITED
a member of the KLUWER ACADEMIC PUBLISHERS GROUP
LANCASTER / BOSTON / THE HAGUE / DORDRECHT

Published in the UK and Europe by
MTP Press Limited
Falcon House
Lancaster, England

British Library Cataloguing in Publication Data

Gresham, G. A.
    Colour atlas of wounds and wounding.
    1. Wounds and injuries — Atlases
    I. Title
    617'.1'0222   RD93

ISBN-13: 978-94-010-8328-7   e-ISBN: 978-94-009-4123-6
DOI: 10.1007/978-94-009-4123-6

Published in the USA by
MTP Press
A division of Kluwer Boston Inc
190 Old Derby Street
Hingham, MA 02043, USA

Library of Congress Cataloging in Publication Data

Gresham, G. A. (Geoffrey Austin)
    Colour atlas of wounds and wounding

    Includes bibliographies and index.
    1. Wounds and injuries.   2. Wounds and injuries — Atlases.
I. Title. [DNLM: 1. Wounds and injuries — atlases. WO 517
G831c]
RD93.G74 1986   617'.1'00222   86-15352
ISBN-13: 978-94-010-8328-7

Phototypesetting by Titus Wilson, Kendal, Cumbria.
Origination and printing by Hartlebury Printers Ltd.,
Kidderminster, Worcs.
Binding by Butler and Tanner Ltd., Frome and London.

CONTENTS

PREFACE

Violence is a steadily increasing feature of modern society caused by devices such as motor vehicles, industrial equipment and aircraft, which are fabricated by man, or caused by man himself. There are few practitioners of medicine who will not encounter wounding in some form in the course of a lifetime of practice. Most wounds will require his skills in treatment; others demand interpretation because the appearance of the wound itself and the pattern in which wounds may be arranged can provide much information about the ways in which they have been caused. For example, the grouping and position of wounds can suggest whether the injuries were inflicted accidentally, suicidally or in the act of homicide. Groups of bruises on a child's body may indicate that injury was not accidental but was inflicted by a parent or other person. In addition, differing appearances of wounds may suggest that they were caused at different times, thus establishing the fact that the assaults were repeated and not a single event.

Earlier definitions of the word suggested that a wound was a breach of the integument of a living thing, either animal or plant. In recent times the term has been broadened to include such things as bruises where the surface of the body is not breached. A more acceptable definition of the wound nowadays would be a lesion caused by mechanical trauma of adequate force, the force required varying with the age and build of the individual and the nature of the implement causing the injury. Slight trauma in the aged can cause extensive bruising whilst having little or no effect on the young person.

This book deals first with the different sorts of wounds, their appearances, methods for determining the age of wounds and so on. The next section deals with patterns of wounding which are important in trying to decide how the wounds might have been caused. The last section is concerned with wounds acquired under different circumstances, such as in vehicular accidents, at work, driving, sporting activities and so on.

When a doctor is called to a scene of death wounds may readily be visible on the corpse. His careful examination and interpretation of the injuries can provide valuable assistance to the police in the early stages of any investigation that may follow. He may be able to say that the wound was self-inflicted, or he may think that the wound had been inflicted homicidally. The events that follow such interpretations are clearly very different so far as the police are concerned. For this, and other reasons, a detailed knowledge of wounds and wounding is an essential part of medical training.

Scientific investigation of the whole subject of trauma has been advancing very slowly over the years. Only in recent times has the matter been pursued with vigour. The Royal College of Pathologists set up a Working Party in 1967 to consider the problem. The aim was to review the state of knowledge in the field of trauma, to assess those areas where knowledge is limited and where advance is required in the interests of basic science and improvement of therapy, and to make recommendations. The report was published in 1972[1]. Not only does it provide a comprehensive review of recent research in the subject but it also indicates those areas where knowledge is lacking, as for example, healing of wounds. This book is written with the suggestions of the Royal College's report well to the fore.

I am grateful to the Chief Constable of Cambridgeshire and the Coroners for the City and County of Cambridge for permission to use some of the pictures. Chris Burton made many of the photographs; his skill has made this work possible. My secretary Susen Green patiently transcribed my manuscript to typescript.

Bibliography

1. *Pathology of Injury: Current Knowledge and Future Development*. (1972). Report of a Working Party of the Royal College of Pathologists, Hunt, A. C. (ed.) (London: Harvey Miller and Medcalf)

Chapter 1

Wounds

Wounds are produced when a mechanical force of one sort or another is applied to the body. The effects produced depend upon the intensity of the applied force and the elastic nature of the tissues. It is the elasticity of the tissues that provides the restoring force that enables the tissue to return to its original form after trauma. However, if the distortion of the tissue exceeds the elastic limit then it will be torn and a wound will be produced.

Wounds vary considerably in appearance. This depends on the shape, density, velocity and weight of the object causing injury and also upon the physical properties of the part of the body traumatized. Every wound, no matter how trivial, must be considered to have some significance and a cause for it must be sought and found. Wounds are often multiple and may be caused by different objects. This is well illustrated by injuries seen in motor vehicle accidents. Such wounds may be caused by bits of glass, blunt prominences in or on the car, and so on (Figure 1.1). Another important point to be borne in mind is that trivial superficial injuries may indicate serious deeper injury which may be due to penetration of vital organs or deeper bruising (Figure 1.2).

Wounds can be classified according to their mode of production:

Ritual
Surgical
Accidental
Suicidal
Homicidal

or they may be classified according to their appearance:

Contusion or bruise
Abrasion
Laceration
Incision
Puncture or stab
Gunshot
Electrical and burns
Patterned

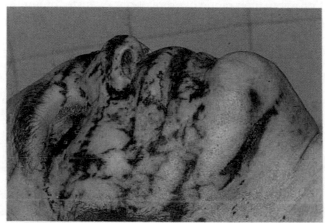

Figure 1.1 *Multiple lacerations and abrasions following impact of the face with a broken car windscreen*

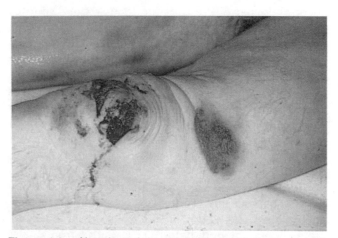

Figure 1.2 *Abrasion of the thigh and lacerations over the knee. Distortion of the limb was due to an extensive comminuted fracture of the lower femur*

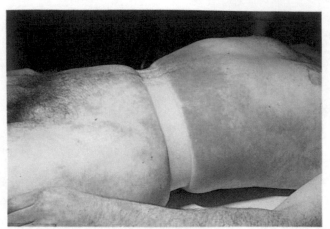

Figure 1.3 *Livor mortis at the back of a body. The pressure of a belt has prevented its development beneath it*

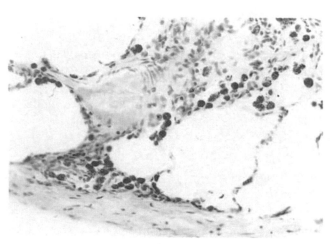

Figure 1.4 *An old bruise of subcutaneous fat showing blue haemosiderin-laden macrophages*

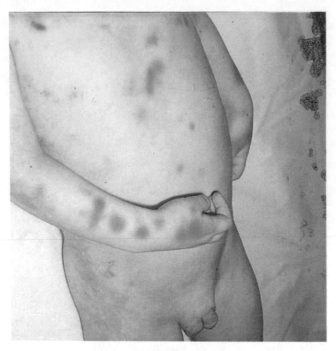

Figure 1.5 *Yellowing bruises on the forearm of a child suggesting injury by fingers gripping the arm*

A contusion, or bruise, is technically speaking not a wound because the surface of the body is often not breached. However, for practical purposes it is included in the category of wounds because its age can be determined more readily than with most wounds. It is usually caused by contact with a blunt object such as a fist, finger-ends, flat pieces of wood, and so on. The force of the blow disrupts small blood vessels which allows blood to leak into the surrounding tissues. Bruises must be distinguished from post-mortem hypostasis or livor mortis. This is a condition due to the seepage of blood into the dependent vessels of a dead body. It takes place about 6 hours after death and unlike a bruise it blanches on pressure. This is because the blood, in livor mortis, is still contained within blood vessels whereas in a bruise the blood has leaked out from the vessels (Figure 1.3).

A bruise changes colour with age so that after 2 or 3 days it has changed from deep purple to a greenish-yellow hue. This is due to the breakdown of haemoglobin from the red blood cells. Ferric iron is also liberated from the haemoglobin and this can be detected by the Prussian blue reaction for haemosiderin. This is done by exposing a section of tissue to potassium ferrocyanide solution and dilute hydrochloric acid. The haemosiderin stains deep blue due to the formation of Prussian blue (Figure 1.4). Haemosiderin can be detected in tissues within 48 hours after bruising; however, the naked-eye colour changes take longer to appear. Whilst it is true that most bruises change in colour with age, those in old people may change very little with the passing of time[1]. Likewise bruises in certain parts of the body, as for example, under the dura, seldom resolve at all. Bruises may also shift with the passage of time thus giving a false impression of the site of injury. For example, a bruise around the hip may gravitate to the tissues around the knee. This is particularly true of deep bruising that may not be readily visible. A detailed dissection can resolve the sequence of events.

Patterns of bruising can often provide useful information about their mode of production. A cluster of bruises on the forearm of a child, each about the size of a finger tip can indicate that the arm was firmly gripped by an assailant (Figure 1.5). In motor vehicle accidents the bruise pattern may be of help in reconstructing the mode of impact of the vehicle with the body.

It is unwise to attempt to deduce the intensity of the injury from the extent of a bruise. Old people and young children tend to bruise more easily than young adults and a boxer can, for example, sustain blows without bruising that would have caused severe bruising in an untrained person. Bruises are modified by a variety of factors. Loose tissues around the eye bruise easily as do tissues that have lost their subcutaneous fat as a result of a wasting disease. This is often a factor in the elderly when the extent of bruising may be out of all

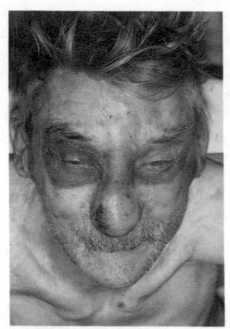

Figure 1.6 *Extensive periorbital bruising following a trivial injury to the nose in an old man*

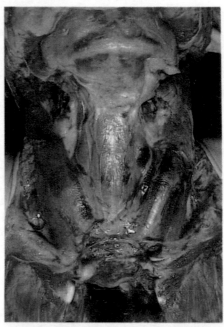

Figure 1.7 *Dissection of anterior neck to show finger bruises due to manual strangulation. The neck had been drained of blood by removing the brain. This prevents post-mortem bruising artefacts in a congested tissue*

proportion to the degree of applied force (Figure 1.6). In general, women tend to bruise more easily than men and those with fair skins display bruises more readily than dark-skinned people. Finally it must not be forgotten that the presence of pre-existing disease, such as thrombocytopenia or hypertension may cause spontaneous bruising or predispose to extensive bruising after minor injuries.

It is true, as a general rule, that bruising does not occur post-mortem. The exception is when severely congested tissues, such as the neck, are traumatized after death. This is particularly important when investigating cases of asphyxia due to manual strangulation. In these circumstances the position and number of finger bruises can be important in determining the mode of asphyxiation. In order to prevent artefactual bruising by dissection of the neck at post-mortem examination it is wise to remove the brain thus allowing blood to drain out of the congested tissues of the head and neck[2] (Figure 1.7).

Abrasions are superficial injuries of the skin where the surface layer of epidermis is rubbed off either by a sliding force as the body travels along a rough surface, or by direct pressure as from a patterned rope round the neck. From the forensic point of view, abrasions, though trivial, are amongst the most informative of wounds. Abrasions can conveniently be subdivided into scratches, grazes and imprint abrasions due to pressure.

Scratches are often seen on the skin after homicidal attack. They occur around the neck following manual strangulation and they are often curved marks reflecting the shape and size of a finger-nail (Figure 1.8). If the

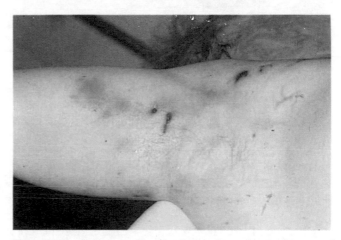

Figure 1.8 *Finger bruises and abrasions due to finger-nail injury in the armpit. Caused by lifting the body after an assault*

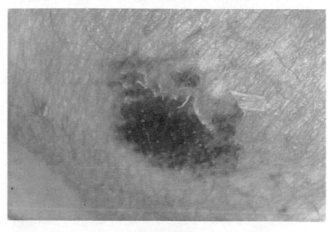

Figure 1.9 *Abrasion showing heaping of the epidermis towards one edge*

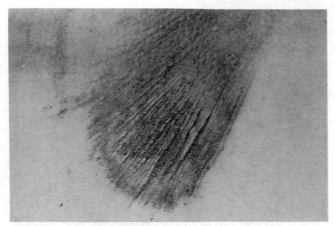

Figure 1.10 *Abrasion showing grit and road tar embedded in the skin*

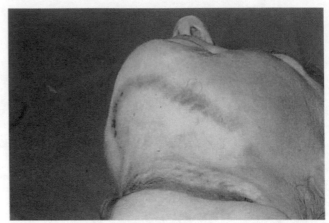

Figure 1.11 *Strangulation with a ligature. The higher mark is abraded and occurred in life. The lower mark is the ligature mark that led to death*

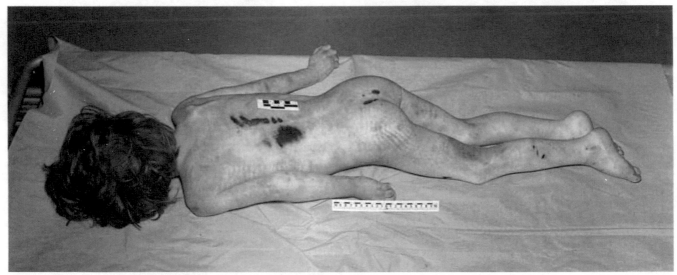

Figure 1.12 *Abrasions caused by the rough leather-covered handle of a whip on a child dead from non-accidental injury*

nail has been drawn across the skin surface the epidermis will form a heap at the finishing edge of the scratch. Similar heaping of epidermis occurs following road traffic injuries and can indicate the direction in which the trauma occurred (Figure 1.9).

Grazes are a form of scratch produced by injury from a rough surface and the pattern of grazing will depend on the nature of the surface. Grazing by gravel produces a coarse pattern whereas that produced by relatively smooth asphalt is less conspicuous (Figure 1.10). Particles of the road surface may be embedded in the graze and the nature of the material may provide an indication of the place of injury. Bitumen from road surfaces varies in composition in different parts of the country and an analysis of the material may furnish useful clues. Many kinds of wounds, apart from abrasions, may have material embedded in them and one must resist the temptation to clean up wounds to get a better view of them before they have been carefully examined for the presence of foreign materials.

Imprint or pressure abrasions are produced by local-ized pressure to the skin. This can be caused by a ligature such as a rope or lanyard (Figure 1.11) or by a whip or stick (Figure 1.12). Various parts of vehicles, such as a radiator grill, leave a characteristic imprint on the skin surface (Figure 1.13) and abrasions are one of the constituents of gunshot wounds when the weapon is discharged at point-blank range causing a rebound impression of the muzzle of the gun on the skin surface (Figure 1.14).

Abrasions can provide much useful information. They can indicate the object that caused them from the material embedded in the wound, the direction of injury, their age from the state of healing and their height from the ground. The position of all wounds should be recorded in relation to the sole of the shod foot if the dead person was wearing shoes. For this purpose the body is marked off in feet from the sole of the shoe and the wounds recorded in relation to these marks (Figure 1.15). Photographic records of any wound should also include a metric scale to record the dimensions of the wound.

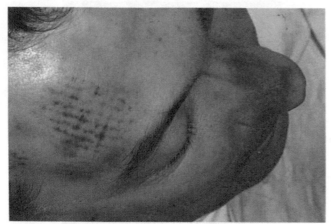

Figure 1.13 *Abrasion of the forehead due to impact with a metal grill*

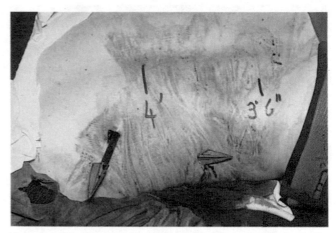

Figure 1.15 *Two wounds produced by cross-bow bolts. Distance from the sole of the foot is marked off on the body in feet and inches*

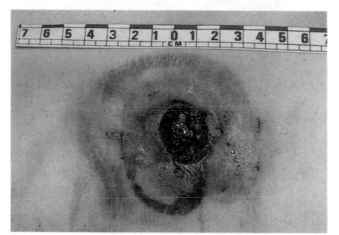

Figure 1.14 *Point-blank discharge of a double-barrelled twelve bore shot-gun. There is an entry hole and an adjacent circular red abrasion caused by the undischarged barrel*

Lacerations are caused by blunt injury of various sorts. They involve splitting of the full thickness of the skin and are often accompanied by bruising and abrasion of the edges of the wound (Figure 1.16). Lacerations tend to be found in places where skin overlies unyielding bone, as for example, the scalp. When they occur elsewhere they are often due to a crushing injury such as a vehicle tyre passing over a leg. Lacerations caused by blunt instruments such as hammers, staves and the like, tend to have a clean sharp edge on one side of the wound which is the point of impact and an opposing ragged edge as the skin rolls away from the weapon. On the scalp this rolling away of the skin may turn the skin flap outwards or inwards. If outwards, hair follicles are often revealed in the depths of the wound (Figure 1.17).

The appearance of the wound varies with the type of instrument that has caused it. Blunt, round-ended objects such as a hammer often produce a stellate laceration in the skin and in the underlying skull following a blow on the head (Figure 1.18). A rod-like weapon on the other hand may produce a linear laceration, the

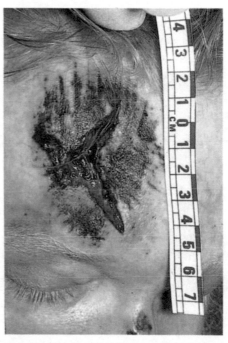

Figure 1.16 *Stellate laceration of the scalp with abrasion of the surrounding skin. Due to a fall from a height onto a height onto a rough concrete surface*

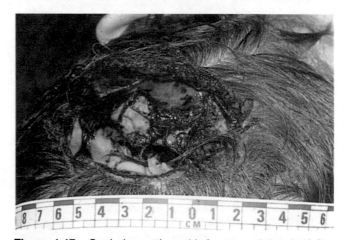

Figure 1.17 *Scalp laceration with fracture of the skull. The edges of the laceration are everted exposing bases of hair follicles*

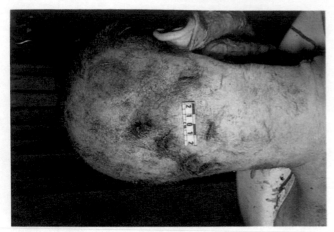

Figure 1.18 *Curved, straight and ragged injuries due to blows with a hammer*

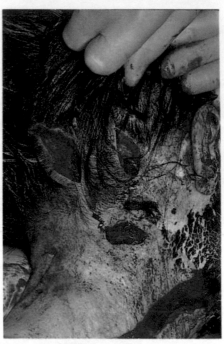

Figure 1.20 *Oval lacerations of the neck behind the ear caused by kicks with the shod foot*

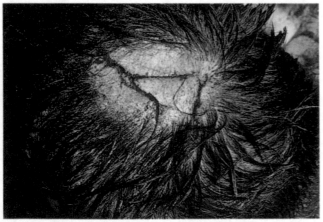

Figure 1.19 *Y-shaped laceration due to a blow on the top of the head with a spanner*

end of which is shaped in the form of a Y (Figure 1.19). Some objects such as the toe cap of a shod foot may produce lacerations that are deceptively like incised wounds. However, careful examination will reveal the features of the wound edges that have previously been described but in addition bridges of unsevered tissue may be seen in the depths of the wound (Figure 1.20) indicating blunt stretching injury rather than incision. In addition, the contour of the toe cap can often be recognized.

In the case of lacerations in particular, the weapon that caused the injury is liable to be contaminated with blood and hair so that samples of blood and hair are regularly collected from the dead person in order to match the materials on the suspected weapon should it be found.

Lacerations of the vagina and perineum are found quite often in rape victims[3]. In addition, lacerations, stab wounds or gunshot wounds may also be found away from the sexual area in these subjects.

Incised wounds are caused by sharp objects such as knives, pieces of glass, axes, and so on. Axe wounds tend to show some bruising of the edges of the wound as well. Incised wounds tend to be longer than deep, unlike lacerations. The edge of the incision is often undercut if the injury was inflicted obliquely and the edges, which are usually sharp, tend to gape. Bleeding is often more profuse than from a laceration because blood vessels are often crushed in the depths of lacerations. However, the edges of an incised wound can be rather ragged as with axe wounds and in loose skin even the sharpest weapon will produce a wound with puckered edges. As with other wounds, bits of the weapon may be found in incisions. Part of the blade may have broken off in the assault and this must be preserved in order to identify the knife. Incised wounds are often found in cases of suicide and homicide.

Stab wounds are caused by penetration of an instrument which may be a sharp knife, a metal rod such as the radio aerial of a car, and the like. The shape and edges of the wound may give indications of the type of knife that has been used. Often, however, repeated stabbing leads to irregularly shaped holes caused by twisting the weapon as it is withdrawn from the body (Figure 1.21). In addition, several stabs may be repeated through the same hole, the weapon not being completely withdrawn from the body. The deepest wound is a guide to the length of the blade, though when pressure is used to force the knife in, tissues may be compressed so that the blade of the knife may be shorter than the deepest wound in the corpse. Some indication of the use of great pressure can be gained by searching the edges of the

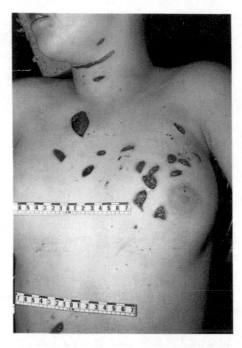

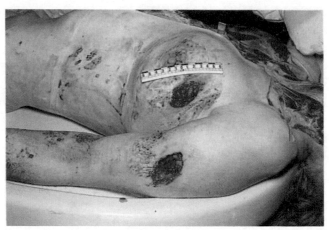

Figure 1.22 *Accidental fatal wounds due to discharge of a 12-bore barrel at about 1 m range. The charge entered the arm, traversed it and entered the chest. The equal size of the arm and chest wounds indicates the close range*

Figure 1.21 *Multiple stab wounds in the upper chest. Some reflect the shape of the blade of the knife, others are irregular in shape due to twisting of the knife on entry or exit from the chest*

wound for bruising or even abrasion. Bruising and abrading of stab wounds is much more likely to occur if the knife has a guard at the base of the blade. Of all wounds, those produced by stabbing may give the least indication from their surface appearance of the serious damage within the body. For example, one stab wound in the neck may penetrate muscle and little else, or may penetrate a major artery producing severe bleeding, or may perforate a large vein producing air embolism.

The question of the degree of force needed to produce stab wounds is often raised. For example, a single homicidal stab wound might be claimed by the defence to be accidental and that the dead person fell on the knife. Clearly, the amount of force needed for such an event would depend upon a number of factors. Experiments with corpses have, to some extent, clarified the position[4]. A spring-loaded knife with a pressure recorder was devised and the cadaver was punctured with it in various ways. The most important fact in the determination of the degree of force needed to effect stabbing was the sharpness of the knife tip. Related to this was the cross-sectional area of the tip of the blade. As little as half a kilogram pressure was needed to penetrate the abdominal skin if the blade tip was pointed, thin and sharp. Clearly then, any view that might be expressed about the degree of force needed to stab with a particular weapon must take into account the state of the weapon at the time of wounding. Much may have happened to that weapon before it is shown as an exhibit in court and an expert witness would do well to make this qualification before expressing any views.

Clothing and the skin itself provide the main resistance to stabbing. Once these have been penetrated little

force is needed to propel the weapon further into the body. Skin that is stretched taut over structures like intercostal spaces or buttocks can be penetrated more easily than floppy abdominal skin, and some parts of the skin are thicker and tougher than others. The velocity of the weapon at the time of impact is important but in most cases this is difficult to assess accurately. These experiments showed quite clearly that if a corpse was allowed to lean forward on to a sharp pointed knife penetration of the body could occur easily. In some circumstances the allegation that the deceased sustained fatal injury by falling on to the point of a knife may well be true.

More will be said about the procedures for the investigation of stab wounds in the section on homicidal wounding (Chapter 3). Knife stabbing has become a serious cause of wounding and homicide in the United Kingdom nowadays. It is a common event in riotous assemblies of gangs of youths and is an increasing cause of injury in domestic disputes.

Gunshot wounds may occur as the result of accident, suicide or homicide (Figure 1.22). The science of ballistics, which is a study of firearms and their ammunition, is a matter for the expert and no pathologist could express more than an elementary view on a mode of shooting. An enormous variety of firearms exists and some are even self-made. Most self-made firearms are used in times of civil strife when supplies of arms may be curtailed.

In most circumstances, however, gunshot wounds will have been caused by small firearms, such as pistols or rifles. These are either smooth-bored or rifled. Smooth-bored are nearly all shot-guns. The internal lining of the barrel is smooth and the diameter of the barrel may be choked at the muzzle. This reduction in size keeps the particles of shot together for a longer period after discharge from the gun than occurs with unchoked weapons. Shot-guns fire cartridges loaded with lead

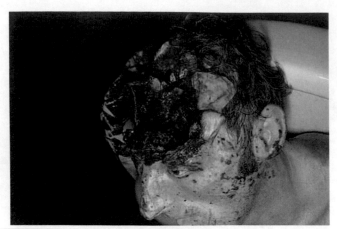

Figure 1.23 *Ragged large exit hole of gunshot wound in the head inflicted with a shot-gun at close range*

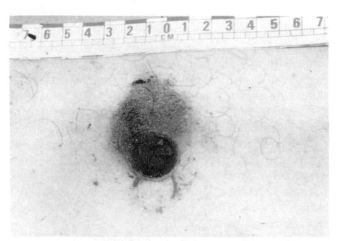

Figure 1.24 *Blackening and burning of the edges of a gunshot wound produced by a 12-bore shot-gun at point-blank range*

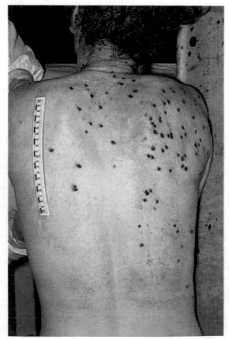

Figure 1.25 *Scatter of shot-gun pellets at a range of about 13 m*

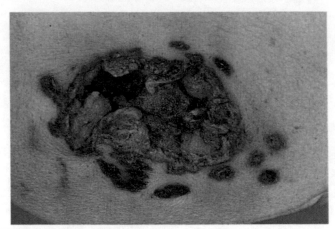

Figure 1.26 *Scatter of shot-gun pellets at 3 m range*

pellets. The shot is enclosed in a cardboard case the base of which is a metal plate. When this is struck by the firing pin of the gun a small prime charge is ignited which then sets off the main propellant charge, which is separated from the lead shot by a pack or wad. Guns of this sort have a range of about 50 m. At close range a wound may show many features due to the various constituents emerging from the muzzle of the gun. These are lead shot, the wad, hot gases and particles of unburned powder. The gunshot wound, at close range, is a compound of various effects such as burning, laceration of skin, tattooing with powder and abrasion if the muzzle recoils against the skin (Figures 1.23, 1.24). If the shot-gun is discharged some distance from the body the lead shot will have scattered and produced a peppering effect on the skin surface (Figure 1.25). The degree of scatter of the shot depends upon the distance of the gun from the body at the time of discharge and the degree of 'choke' on the muzzle. In general, marginal pellet holes are seen with a range of about 2 m (Figure 1.26). Further away the degree of spread in centimetres is about three times the distance away of the gun, in metres.

Rifled weapons have spiral grooves running along the internal length of the barrel. This impresses a distinctive mark on the metal case of the bullet as it rotates at speed down the barrel. Such weapons have a greater range than shot-guns and the missile may travel 1000 m or more.

In cases of shooting it is often necessary to determine the entry and exit holes of the missiles. With shot-gun injuries this is not difficult. At close range the entry hole is comparatively small showing the features already described. The exit hole, if present, is on the other hand large and ragged (Figure 1.27). If the wound is to the head pieces of brain and bone may be expelled from the ragged exit hole and lie scattered about the area.

Exit and entry holes are not always so easily identified following wounds with high velocity rifled weapons. A bullet leaving the muzzle of a pistol will have a degree of tail-wag on it up to about 50 m; after this it settles down to a true 'nose-on' course[5]. The result of this is

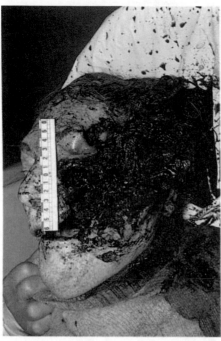

Figure 1.27 *Large exit hole in the skull and face following suicidal shooting by discharging the gun with the muzzle placed in the mouth*

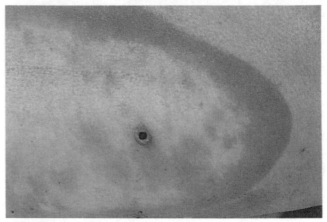

Figure 1.28 *Entry hole of high velocity bullet showing everted edges*

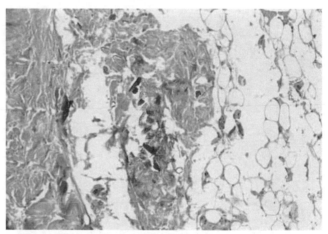

Figure 1.29 *Histological section of entry hole of high velocity bullet showing green material from the bullet in the subcutaneous tissue*

that at close range the entry hole of a high velocity bullet may have a frayed edge whereas the exit hole may have a edge that is sharply defined (Figure 1.28). This latter depends upon the structures that the missile encounters as it passes through the body. If it strikes hard bone its speed will be greatly reduced and the exit hole will be large and ragged, particularly if bits of bone leave the body through the hole.

If there is doubt about the distinction between entry and exit holes of high velocity missiles it can often be resolved by careful examination of the wounds by naked eye and microscopy. As the bullet enters it wipes material from its surface on to the skin, which can be seen easily or can be demonstrated in histological sections (Figure 1.29).

Electrical wounds are usually accidental or suicidal. As with ballistic injury the help of an expert is needed in interpreting the likely effects of an electrical injury. They depend upon many factors, such as the nature of the current (a.c. or d.c.), frequency, voltage, amperage, duration of application of the current, whether the body was effectively earthed (e.g. by wet feet) and, above all, the path of the current through the body. If the current passed from arm to arm across the chest the chances of fatal cardiac arrest are high. Most of this information is available if the domestic supply of electricity is involved. But with an event such as a strike of lightning, very little evidence of the intensity of the electrical force is available.

Alternating currents produce tetanic contractions of muscle so that the individual will have difficulty in releasing the point of contact. Voltages as low as 100

volts may be fatal, whereas individuals may survive a single shock of 10 000 volts. At low voltages the cause of death is usually a cardiac arrest whereas at higher voltage electrothermal injury plays a part. Essentially the outcome of the electrical contact, which depends upon the amperage, varies with the resistance of the body tissues. Electrical accidents can be classified according to amperage into four main groups[6]. As a general rule 30 mA is the tolerance limit, 40 mA will produce unconsciousness and 100 mA produce death.

The skin is the most electrically resistant part of the body particularly the thick skin of the palms, hands, scalp and back of the body. Excessive sweating due to heat, fever or drugs that induce sweating makes the skin much less resistant to the passage of the current. Rubber gloves and leather soles, provided they do not have metal nails or toe caps, will provide adequate protection.

A good deal of experimental work done on animals has indicated that sudden death from electrocution is usually due to a cardiac dysrhythmia, such as ventricular

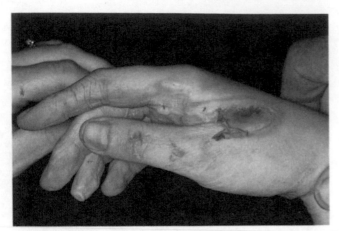

Figure 1.30 *Electrical injury with parchment-like skin in the centre and a zone of hyperaemia at the edge*

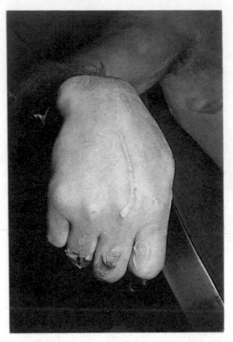

Figure 1.32 *Linear blistering in an electrical injury*

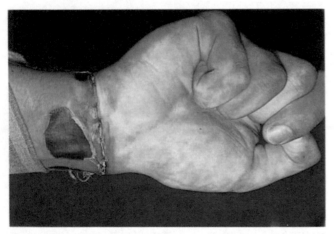

Figure 1.31 *Suicidal electrocution showing parchment-like burn with raised edges and erythema in the proximal side of the arm and the wrist*

fibrillation, or from injury to the brainstem with suppression of the activity of the respiratory and other centres.

The external features of electrical injury are so-called 'current' marks that occur at the points of entry and exit of the electrical discharge. They are not always readily visible if cutaneous resistance is reduced or if the duration of contact is very short. Furthermore, if the current is applied over a large area of the body, current marks are not seen. A particular example of this is electrocution of a body immersed in a bath of water.

The main factor in producing a current mark is heat; this occurs within the tissue but external burning can also contribute to the mark if the clothing ignites as well. As with other burns a zone of hyperaemia or even vesiculation may be seen around the current mark (Figures 1.30, 1.31, 1.32). Negatively charged ions are also produced in tissues by electrolysis and these combine with the metal of the electrical contact to form

metal salts that are deposited in the tissues. In addition, cells are elongated and forced apart by the passage of the current so that gaps occur between cells. These are called electric channels.

Current marks can be induced post-mortem and they closely resemble the current marks produced in life. Detection of a vital reaction is necessary to distinguish ante-mortem and post-mortem electrical damage.

Lightning injury, though rare, is one of the most extreme forms of electrical injury in that current peaks of up to 200 000 amps and 20 million volts can be generated. About 12 people each year are struck by lightning in the UK and about 150 in the USA. These strikes occur mainly during 'dry thunderstorms', perhaps because cloud-to-ground lightning strikes are more often encountered under these circumstances. The lightning strike is a complex discharge, first with a leader from ground to cloud or cloud to ground. This is followed by a main return stroke along the same path but in the opposite direction and there may be as many as 40 peaks of current of the magnitude previously described.

The effects upon the person, as with other electrical injuries, are a compound of the electrical and thermal discharges. The injuries include damage to skin and clothing, arborescent burns, fractured bones due to blast and metallic articles on the person which may become magnetized. The blast effect of the discharge may also cause contusions of the heart, lungs and gut and cerebral oedema, due to brainstem damage, may develop rapidly if the individual survives[7]. Other neurological diseases may appear if the person survives: they include amnesia, reversible flaccid paralysis, as well as

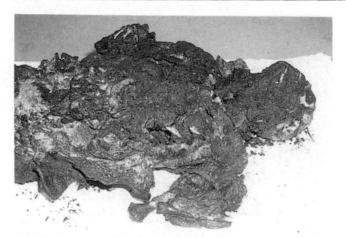

Figure 1.33 *Severe charring and destruction of a body by fire*

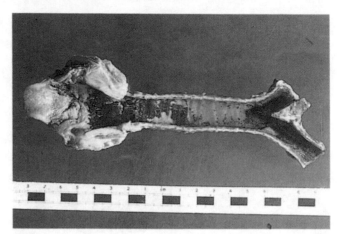

Figure 1.35 *Tongue, trachea and main bronchi showing soot in the air passages indicating that breathing occurred whilst the burning took place*

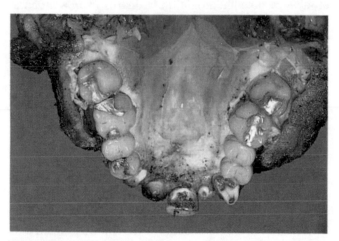

Figure 1.34 *Upper jaw of a burned corpse. The front teeth have been fractured by heat but the rear teeth are well preserved and are valuable for identification*

a variety of spastic paralyses[8]. It is well to remember that vigorous attempts at resuscitation should be continued if cardiorespiratory arrest occurs. It has been suggested that these patients can withstand apnoea for some time because the electrical effect halts cellular metabolism and thereby delays the injurious effect of hypoxia when cardiorespiratory arrest has occurred.

Burning is one of the components of electrical injury but it can obviously occur in other ways. As a cause of death burns are usually accidentally induced as a result of fires in domestic circumstances. Severe burning can also occur as a result of explosions or vehicle accidents when the automobiles involved burst into flames. They are a regular feature of deaths from aircraft accidents[9].

Burns may be relatively trivial or superficial when some of the skin elements remain after burning. Deep burns involve the whole dermal layer and vary from surface injury to total disintegration of the part of the body involved. The mechanism of tissue damage is principally thermal although other features play a part. Fluid is readily lost from damaged blood vessels which exude plasma into the tissues. This is the result of endothelial destruction and also endothelial cell contraction caused by vasotropic substances in the burn; one of these is histamine. Endothelial contraction produces interendothelial gaps through which plasma escapes into the burned area. This leakage of plasma leads to local haemoconcentration in blood vessels and sludging of erythrocytes, which in turn predisposes to thrombosis. The effects of this are to increase the extent of damage around the area of burning[10].

Burns in confined spaces, such as rooms, caravans and the like, are often severe because the person may have been overcome by carbon monoxide produced by the incomplete burning of clothing, pillows, furniture and so on. Sometimes the body may be totally destroyed by heat and all that remains are a few fragments of charred broken bones and teeth. Occasionally in paralysed or infirm persons, seated in chairs, burning may be confined to the torso and the legs and arms drop off and remain recognizable (Figure 1.33). Once ignited the human body burns like a candle; the subcutaneous fat melts and burns fiercely. Burning is a most effective way of destroying a body so that every attempt should be made at the scene to recover every fragment of the body that might be of value in identification of the person. The teeth are of great importance in this regard (Figure 1.34). It is also important to establish whether the individual was alive at the time the fire occurred because they may have been killed beforehand and then burnt. The presence of soot in the air passages (Figures 1.35, 1.36), and of carboxyhaemoglobin in the blood support the view that the person was alive when

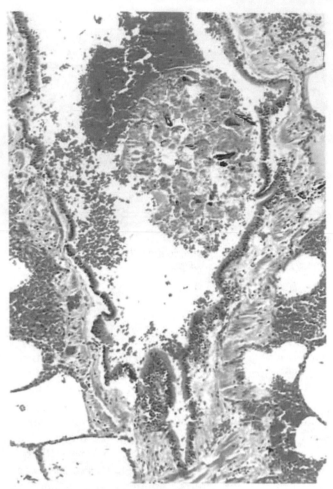

Figure 1.36 *Section of lung showing carbon particles in a bronchiole*

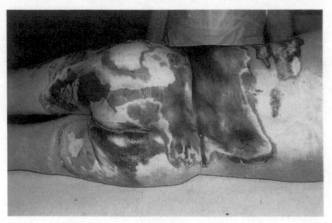

Figure 1.38 *A burn caused by hot liquid which subsequently ignited. The burn occurred a few days before death. A bright red inflammatory reaction has developed at the edges of the burn*

the fire took place. It is common to find blood levels of 40% carboxyhaemoglobin in deaths from accidental burning.

Burns from moist heat, such as steam and hot liquids, are confined to the surface of the body, either the skin or mucous membranes. The severe deeper injury produced by dry heat is rarely seen in such cases (Figures 1.37, 1.38). Other sorts of burns are produced by corrosive chemicals. These vary in colour according to the nature of the chemical involved. Nitric acid produces a brown burn whereas those produced by hydrochloric and sulphuric acids are reddish-black. Phenol causes white areas of skin destruction. Certain ointments containing phenolic substances when applied to the sensitive thin skin of infants, can cause areas of skin damage. These need to be distinguished from burns inflicted as a result of non-accidental injury.

Patterned wound is a term used to describe wounds which indicate by their pattern and situation on the body whether death was the result of accident, suicide or homicide. Several kinds of wound often make up the pattern. For example, in manual strangulation there may be a combination of a pressure abrasion due to the ligature, curved finger-nail marks caused either by the assailant or the victim struggling to release the ligature, and bruises (Figure 1.39). Patterned wounds will form an important part of the sections dealing with accident, suicide and homicide (Chapter 3). There are, however, two sorts that can be dealt with now.

Bite marks may be inflicted by man or other animals. They have received a good deal of attention in recent times because of their occurrence in child victims of non-accidental injury. However, they occur in other forms of homicide and have been well recognized for at least the past 50 years. The assessment of bite wounds and the precise identification of the person who produced them is the specialized field of the forensic odontologist of whom there are very few in the United

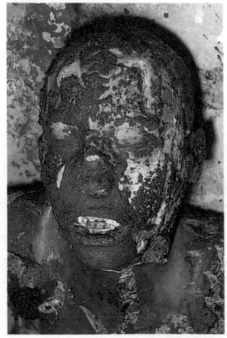

Figure 1.37 *Severe charring due to dry heat. The features are largely destroyed but the teeth are preserved*

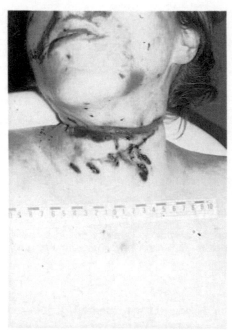

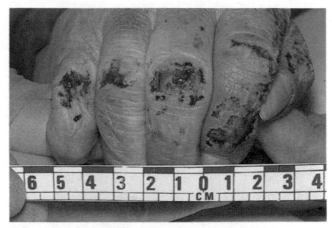

Figure 1.40 *Rat bites of the fingers inflicted after death*

Figure 1.39 *A pattern of wounding showing a ligature mark on the neck, a bruise on the jaw above and superficial stab wounds made with pointed scissors below the ligature*

Kingdom[11]. Bite marks are a combination of bruising, abrasion and laceration. In the abused children they are often faint and difficult to see and ultraviolet photography might be required in order to show them clearly[12]. An interesting feature of such bite marks is that the initial lesion may fade away to become visible a few months after injury. The likely explanation for this is that melanocytes tend to migrate slowly to the edges of wounds and they indicate their presence by absorbing ultraviolet light, so that the wounds can only be demonstrated when a sufficient quantity of melanocytes has collected at the edges.

Bite marks in other sorts of homicide are often more clearly defined and look as though they were inflicted more slowly and deliberately than in the childhood cases. This may be because they were inflicted as part of a sexual act. Photography of bite marks by ordinary and ultraviolet light is essential and a metric scale should be included in the photograph. Bite marks on the skin or in deeper structures should be carefully swabbed with a swab moistened in distilled water in order to detect any saliva that might be present. This will enable blood group substances to be found and identified. However, because 80% of the population secrete blood group substances in their saliva and other body fluids it is important to swab the bite mark from the edge towards the centre in order to avoid contamination by the sweat of the individual who has been bitten.

If the skin is pierced the bite may become infected with a variety of organisms that are often resistant to many antibiotics. Related to bites are tooth wounds of the hands and knuckles that may be found on the assailant. These wounds also become infected because

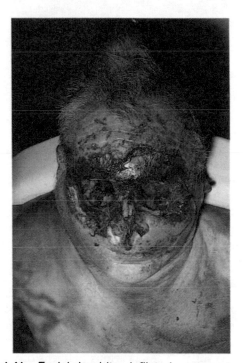

Figure 1.41 *Facial dog bites inflicted post-mortem*

mouth organisms are well embedded in the tissues as the result of fighting. If the joints are pierced arthritis, ankylosis and septicaemia can result. It is interesting to note that one quarter of all hand infections seen at the Sacramento Medical Centre were caused by tooth injuries following a fight[13].

Animal bites rarely present a problem in diagnosis for the forensic pathologist. They are most often seen as post-mortem injuries on dead bodies caused by rats, fish, dogs, foxes and the like, when the body has not been found for some days after death (Figures 1.40, 1.41). Occasionally multiple puncture holes may be mistaken for stab wounds[14]. The problem can be resolved by a detailed examination of the wounds followed by dental impressions. The discovery of dental calculus, epithelial squamous cells and bacteria by microscopic

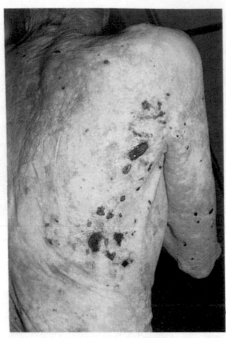

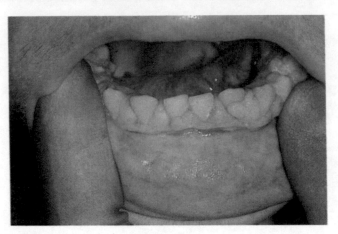

Figure 1.43 *Hypertrophy of the gums in an epileptic child that had been treated for a long time with diphenylhydantoin*

Figure 1.42 *Abrasion produced by self-scratching (dermatitis artefacta). The lesions occur in areas that can be reached by the subject's hands*

examination of the contents of the wounds can also be of assistance in diagnosis.

Injuries caused by wild animals are not an uncommon part of the work of the doctor in tropical areas. They vary in appearance according to the type of animal that has inflicted the wound. Snake bites, which usually occur on the dorsum of the foot, show two small puncture holes if a cobra has bitten. More closely set smaller bites, in pairs, can be caused by centipedes whereas a single puncture is the result of the sting in the tail of scorpions. Monkey bites are often superficial but there may be a good deal of scratching of the adjacent skin surfaces as well[15]. These various patterns of wounding soon come to be recognized by the physician, indeed the pattern of a crocodile bite, in an individual who survived, is most dramatic.

Self-inflicted wounds form a series of patterns which require recognition if effective therapy is to be instituted. Self-destructive behaviour may take the form of suicide or focal injury and is a manifestation of a primary aggressive tendency directed against one's self. It may occur as a result of a psychiatric illness or malingering, or as an erotic motive. There are several other complex reasons for this form of injury referred to by some as 'focal suicide'[16]. Prisoners and persons in mental hospitals may use focal injury as a form of protest: severance of the Achilles tendon, razor blade, glass and wood injuries are examples. Neurotic patients usually attack their skin by pinching, scratching, biting, plucking out of hair, and so on. There are some familial diseases associated with self-mutilation, such as the Lesch–Nyhan syndrome which is a disorder of uric acid

metabolism associated with mental deficiency and destructive biting of the lips.

Ritual wounds come into this class. Though not self-inflicted these mutilations are acceptable to those who wish to follow certain religions. The religions of Islam and Judaism, and many native tribes about the world, have such rites. All sorts of mutilations are practised such as foot binding, ear and nose piercing and lip splitting, teeth filing, ritual circumcision of women, and so on. In the past women of the Amazon had their breasts amputated so that they could be more effective in battle. Being without a breast is the origin of the word Amazon.

The skin is a favourite target area for self-mutilation and damage may vary from minor excoriations and scars to severe injuries, such as amputations. Broadly speaking, there are three main sorts of self-injury:

(1) Neurotic excoriation
(2) Delusions of parasitism
(3) Factitial dermatitis

Neurotic excoriations are small superficial ulcers which heal by scarring and adjacent pigmentation (Figure 1.42). The chest, sides of arms, legs and face are often involved and left-sided lesions are more often found in right-handed persons. The patient who believes he has parasites attempts to destroy them by scratching, the use of instruments or by the application of caustic substances. Repeated application of caustics may cause lesions that mimic well-established skin conditions such as psoriasis. Only when the patient applies an excess of the caustic which then trickles along the skin to produce a tell-tale line is the cause suspected[17].

The patient with factitial dermatitis denies all knowledge of the cause of the condition. Lesions suddenly appear in a bizarre arrangement, the patient complaining of a sensation of a burrowing in the skin beforehand. A variety of instruments and chemicals may be used to produce the lesions and cigarette burning is frequent.

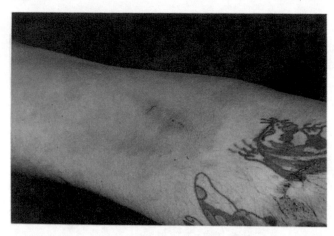

Figure 1.44 *Purple streaks in the skin of ante-cubital fossa are thrombosed veins caused by repeated injections*

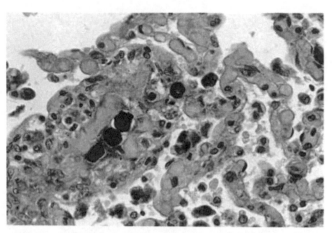

Figure 1.46 *Section of lung stained by the PAS method showing magenta-coloured granules of corn starch in pulmonary capillaries. The section was taken from a drug addict who died of methadone poisoning*

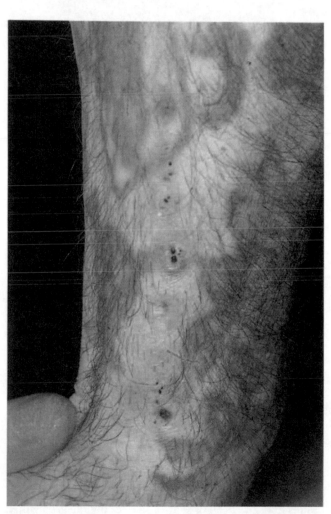

Figure 1.45 *Punched-out 'pop ulcers' caused by extravasation of barbiturates into the skin following inexpert injection*

Many sorts of lesions may be seen varying from ulcers, tattoo marks from the injection of materials into the skin, hypertrophic scars due to repeated rubbing of buttocks, elbows and so on. These are particularly seen in epileptics treated with the drug diphenylhydantoin (Figure 1.43). Injections of milk, air, faecal material and drugs have all been recorded. Milk gives a Weber–Christian-like syndrome, air produces subcutaneous emphysema and faecal material causes localized abscesses and septicaemia. Injection of drugs by addicts is a form of self-destructive behaviour. Attempted intravenous injections of heroin or barbiturate tablets ground up and suspended in dirty water, often from a lavatory pan, cause repeated thrombosis of superficial veins (Figure 1.44). 'Skin-popping' which is the subcutaneous injection of drugs, such as barbiturates, may lead to punched-out areas of ulceration closely resembling those that used to be seen in chrome salt workers in industry (Figure 1.45). Sharing of syringes promotes serum hepatitis and endocarditis is also the result of intravenous injection of bacteria. Foreign materials, such as starch granules from intravenously injected tablets may be found on microscopy of the lung. The particles are seen in capillaries and some foreign particles evoke a widespread granulomatous response throughout the lung leading to disorders of gas diffusion (Figure 1.46). A useful aid in the post-mortem examination of the drug addict is to pass a quantity of blood through a millipore filter. If this is then stained by the PAS method magenta-coloured starch granules may be found in the filtrate. This indicates the vast amounts of such materials that are sometimes injected intravenously.

Sexual mutilation of various kinds is seen. Sometimes the genitals are amputated or part of the genital apparatus, such as a testis, is cut off. Self-induced vaginal wounds may present as vaginal bleeding[18], repeated

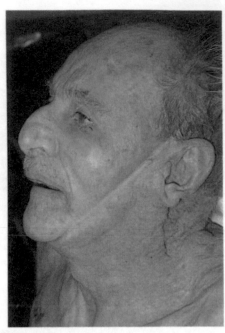

Figure 1.47 *Typical linear mark produced after death by a bandage to keep the mouth closed. No evidence of any swelling or vital reaction at the edges of the post-mortem injury*

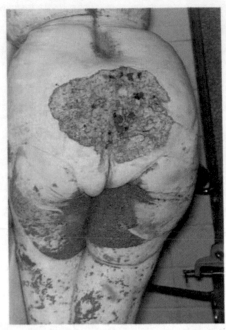

Figure 1.48 *Extensive loss of skin over the sacrum. This is due to post-mortem bites by rats in a drowned person recovered from the river after some days*

urethral trauma with sticks, rubber tubes and the like may cause a stricture, and so on.

Certain syndromes are associated with self-inflicted injury. Polysurgery, or a compulsion to submit to surgical operations is a form of attempted self-destruction. The abdominal wall of such people is often likened to a battle-ground because of the multiple surgical scars. Munchausen's syndrome, named after the hero of German folklore, Baron von Munchausen, who was famed for his tales of fantasy and exaggeration, occurs in people who have often had relations with physicians in their youth. The physician becomes the focal point of life and the patients use all sorts of medical and paramedical devices to secure attention. Purposeful accidents form yet another syndrome of attempted self-destruction by trains, cars, falls from heights, and so on.

Determination of the age of wounds is often of considerable forensic importance. Wounds that are inflicted after death show no evidence of a vital reaction. For example, a tight bandage placed under the chin of a corpse and tied over the head to keep the mouth closed will sometimes produce a parchment-like mark along the side of the face (Figure 1.47). If the body is bumped after death, being brought down narrow stairs for example, parchment-like clearly defined marks may be found over the body. It is important to distinguish these from ante-mortem injury. If a corpse has been floating for some time in rivers or at sea severe post-mortem injury may result from collision with boats and bridges. In addition, extensive animal bites by fish or rats may be

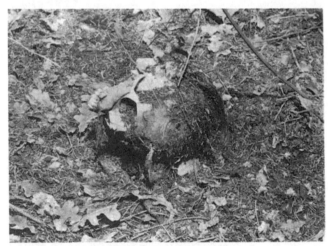

Figure 1.49 *Skull detached from the body of a dead girl. It had probably been torn off the body by a fox and deposited some distance away from the rest of the corpse*

found (Figure 1.48). Larger predators, such as foxes, may dismember a body (Figure 1.49). The neck organs are torn out and the head or limbs may also become detached from the body in this way. Much of the soft tissues may be eaten or scattered over a wide area which makes identity difficult sometimes and eliminates the possibility of establishing some causes of death, such as asphyxia due to mechanical constriction of the neck.

It is important to appreciate the fact that multiple wounds on a body may not all have been produced at the same time. For example, death may be caused by a stab wound and then the dead body is placed on a railway line. Determining the age of wounds is not always easy particularly when they have been inflicted shortly before death. Furthermore, wounds in different tissues do not heal at the same rate: most of the experimental work on the subject has been done on the skin and this must be borne in mind when interpreting results. Wounds are biochemically asymmetrical in that the levels of PO_2 and pH are low in the active margins in the first few days of healing[19]. So it is that local and systemic factors may greatly influence the rate of wound healing. For example, collagen formation in wounds may be delayed in many systemic disorders such as hypoxia, hypovolaemia, dehydration, hypothermia, multiple trauma, and so on. Chronic disease states such as uraemia, neoplasia, sepsis elsewhere in the body and vitamin C and zinc deficiencies may also delay wound healing. Local factors such as haematoma, sepsis and foreign bodies are well-known factors that influence wound strength[20].

Many attempts have been made to determine the age of wounds within a few hours of death and the matter is fully reviewed by Raekallio[21]. Naked-eye examination of wounds such as abrasions and bruises can often afford an indication of the age of the wound. This gives only a crude estimate. A graze is usually red and swollen at the edges about 12 h after the injury and this is about the earliest interval that can be assessed by visual examination. Bleeding from a wound can occur post-mortem in congested tissues and blood clots after death so that the finding of fibrin in the wound is no indication of its ante-mortem origin. Microscopic examination of the wound is an essential part of the assessment and gives an opportunity to recognize the age of wounds inflicted near to death. For example, pavementing of leukocytes along the endothelial cells of blood vessels and their extravasation into the adjacent tissues are seen a few hours after wounding. The precise time is much debated by various workers ranging from 4 to 24 h. To some extent the discrepancy between different workers is related to their definition of what is meant by a distinct leukocytic infiltration.

However, ordinary light microscopy is of no value in the assessment of the age of a wound inflicted within 4 h of death of the subject. For this purpose histochemical reactions for the detection of enzymes and vasoactive substances released as a result of the inflammatory reaction are necessary. These and other methods will now be described in relation to the various sorts of wounds that we have already considered.

Open skin injuries include lacerations, abrasions, incised and stab wounds. Early work with these lesions concentrated on a study of the staining properties of connective tissue fibres in the wounds. It was said that Mallory's stain, containing acid fuchsin and aniline blue, stained connective tissue fibres differently according to whether they had been produced ante-mortem or post-mortem. However, the demonstration of staining properties of such fibres in tissues after rigor mortis had subsided and which resembled ante-mortem staining rendered the use of this method invalid. Likewise refraction and aggregation of elastic fibres, which was said to be a feature of ante-mortem wounds, was later shown post-mortem[22].

A number of acid glycosaminoglycans have been examined in skin wounds by histochemical methods. These substances decrease in amount in a zone of the wound close to its edge about 32 h after injury. It is said that they do not alter in strangulation wounds produced ante-mortem.

Up to the fifth day after wounding there is an increase in the level of acid aminoglycans in the wound. This is obviously of no value in determining the early age of wounds but is useful in ageing the sorts of wounds found in children that have been injured non-accidentally. Such methods enable one to establish evidence of repeated, rather than a single injury. Likewise the detection of RNA in increased amounts in regenerating fibroblasts is maximal at about 8 days after wounding and it starts to increase about 32 h after death.

In recent times histochemical methods for the study of enzymes in wounds have been employed. For both histological and histochemical purposes the wound is excised with about 1 cm of the surrounding tissue. Half is fixed in 10% formalin at 4 °C overnight. This piece is used for the demonstration of phosphatases and esterases and for routine histological purposes. The other piece is frozen in liquid nitrogen for the demonstration of aminopeptidases and adenosinetriphosphatases. Decreased enzyme activity occurs in the central zone of the wound which is a zone about 500 μm wide midway between the edge and deeper parts of the wound. On the other hand, the deeper peripheral part of the wound shows increased enzymatic activity. Such changes do not occur in post-mortem wounds and can therefore be considered to be part of a vital reaction to injury. The various enzyme changes take place at different times so enabling a sort of biological timetable to be constructed. These changes then persist for up to about 5 days. Esterases and ATPase increase at about 2 h in the peripheral zone. Acid and alkaline phosphatases increase at 4 and 8 h respectively. This increase of enzymes in the more peripheral parts of the wound probably reflects synthesis by adjacent viable cells as a prelude to healing[23].

Another approach to the problem of timing wounds is the measurement of histamine, serotonin and other vasoactive amines in the wound. For this purpose about 2 g of injured skin and adjacent control tissue is extracted and the amine estimated spectrofluorimetrically. Studies have been done on strangulation marks when the time of death was precisely known and also on injured skin in guinea-pigs. In about 30 min after wounding free histamine levels are maximal whereas serotonin appears early, in about 10 min. The reaction tends to be biphasic in that a further rise of serotonin occurs about 2 h later. Estimations of noradrenaline have also been used but this substance disappears rap-

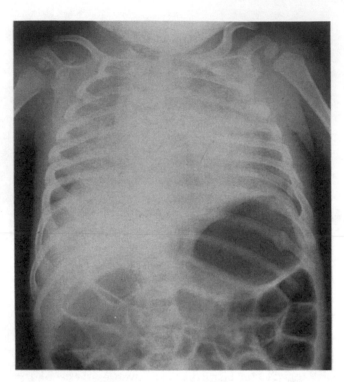

Figure 1.50 *Swelling of a lower left rib due to fracture callus. The healing fracture can be clearly seen in the gas shadow of the stomach in the right of the picture*

idly after the death of the subject and is consequently of limited value. The later stages of the healing process have been extensively studied and reviewed. In general, the greater the degree of differentiation of a tissue the slower is the healing process[24].

The age of bruises can also be assessed by histological and histochemical methods. Bruises are caused by extravasation of blood into the tissues and must be differentiated from artefacts that can be produced in the neck organs for example, by post-mortem dissection. Downward traction on neck organs in their removal from the body will produce extravasation of blood into the deep tissues in a large proportion of the cases[25]. Careful dissection and drainage of blood by prior removal of the brain will prevent these artefacts which cannot be distinguished easily from ante-mortem bruising.

Haemosiderin appears in a bruise at about 48 h after bruising but haematoidin takes about 9 days to appear. Enzyme changes in bruises broadly reflect those seen in other wounds.

The presence of a visible vital reaction at the edges of burns provides evidence of an ante-mortem origin. Vesiculation of burns is usually an ante-mortem phenomenon, particularly if leukocytes and fibrin are found in the vesicles. It has, however, been reported that vesicles can also appear in a burn shortly after death[26]. Enzyme methods have not been used on human material in the ageing of burns. Electrical burns cannot be distinguished from burns of other sorts on histologi-

cal examination. The presence of current channels and nuclear elongation may assist in distinguishing electrical burns but these appearances are also seen as a result of freezing of tissues as in frost-bite. Most current marks contain metallic fragments which can be demonstrated by histochemical methods or by scanning electron microscopy of samples taken from the wound with a moist applicator. Metals such as aluminium, copper, iron and zinc have been found and these help to distinguish electrical from other burns.

Determination of the ages of bony fractures is a matter of some importance because fractures are a common feature of the non-accidental injury syndrome in children. Establishing the fact that fractures are of different ages can be important in supporting the view that the child had been injured repeatedly. The following histological sequences have been described in the healing of fractures[27]:

(1) Many polymorphonuclear leukocytes appear in the fracture line at about 4 h after injury and from 1 to 8 h extravasated blood and the inflammatory exudate develop.

(2) Within the first week spicules of bone arranged in an irregular woven pattern form around blood vessels. This is the first new bone formation and it is laid down by abundant osteoblasts which elaborate phosphatase as early as 10 h after injury. The new woven bone forms a knob at the fracture line. This is called primary callus and the fracture can be readily seen in a radiograph (Figure 1.50).

(3) The primary callus is gradually removed and replaced by mature lamellar bone laid down along stress lines in the bone. This reconstruction of the form of the bone to its original shape may take as long as a year to occur.

The rate of future healing is influenced by the general and local factors that have already been described for the healing of other wounds. In children the formation of primary callus is often exuberant and the cellular activity is so great in the area of repair that it may be confused with a malignant neoplasm when viewed under the microscope. Movement also has a powerful influence. Total immobilization of a fracture will delay healing but excessive movement will also prevent healing and lead to the formation of a pseudoarthrosis or false joint between the broken ends. The joint may develop cartilaginous surfaces and it is interesting that cartilage formation is also a feature of mobile fractures such as those in the ribs, even though a pseudoarthrosis has not formed. This cartilage is ultimately turned to bone by the process of endochondral ossification. Much of the new bone found in fractures arises however from formation of bone in membrane – membranous ossification.

In Courts of Law the pathologist is often pressed to give a precise opinion upon the age of a wound. All he can do is to enunciate the principles of the methods available for determining wound age and to sound a note of caution about the many, often ill-defined, variables that may affect the healing process in a particular case.

Bibliography

1. Camps, F. E. (1952). Interpretation of wounds. *Br. Med. J.*, **2**, 770
2. Gresham, G. A. (1978). Violent forms of asphyxial death. In Mason, J. K. (ed.) *The Pathology of Violent Injury*. (London: Edward Arnold)
3. Everett, R. B. and Jimerson, G. K. (1977). The rape victim. A review of 117 consecutive cases. *Obstet. Gynaecol.*, **50**, 88
4. Knight, B. (1975). The dynamics of stab wounds. *Forensic Sci.*, **6**, 249
5. Simpson, K. (1979). Fire-arm wounds. In *Forensic Medicine*, 8th Edn. (London: Edward Arnold)
6. Koeppen, S. (1961). Der Elektrische Unfall. *Elektromedizin*, **6**, 215
7. Leader. (1974). Lightning. *Br. Med. J.*, **2**, 181
8. Sharma, M. and Smith, A. (1978). Paraplegia as a result of lightning injury. *Br. Med. J.*, **2**, 1464
9. Mason, J. K. (1978). The aircraft accident as an example of a major disaster. In Mason, J. K. (ed.) *The Pathology of Violent Injury*. (London: Edward Arnold)
10. Sevitt, S. (1970). Reflections of some problems in the pathology of trauma. *J. Trauma*, **10**, 962
11. Harvey, W. (ed.) (1976). *Dental Identification and Forensic Odonotology*. (London: Henry Kimpton)
12. Ruddick, R. F. (1974). A technique for recording bite marks for forensic studies. *Med. Biol. Illust.*, **24**, 128
13. Leader. (1977). Tooth wounds and the infected fist. *Lancet*, **2**, 341
14. Glass, R. T., Jordan, F. B. and Andrews, E. E. (1975). Multiple animal bite wounds. A case report. *J. Forensic Sci.*, **20**, 305
15. Shattock, F. M. (1968). Injuries caused by wild animals. *Lancet*, **2**, 412
16. Eckert, W. G. (1977). The pathology of self-mutilation and destructive acts: a forensic study and review. *J. Forensic Sci.*, **22**, 242
17. Sneddon, I. and Sneddon, J. (1975). Self-inflicted injury: a follow-up study of 43 patients. *Br. Med. J.*, **2**, 527
18. Carney, M. W. P. and Brozovic, M. (1978). Self-inflicted bleeding and bruising. *Lancet*, **1**, 924
19. Hunt, T. K. and Pai, M. P. (1972). The effect of varying ambient oxygen tensions on wound metabolism and collagen synthesis. *Surg. Gynaecol. Obstet.*, **135**, 561
20. Leader. (1973). To heal the wound. *Lancet*, **1**, 84
21. Raekallio, J. (1973). Estimation of the age of injuries by histochemical and biochemical methods. *Z. Rechtsmed.*, **73**, 83
22. Fatteh, A. (1971). Distinction between ante-mortem and post-mortem wounds: a study of elastic fibres in human skin. *J. Forensic Sci.*, **16**, 393
23. Pullar, P. (1973). The histopathology of wounds. In Mant, K. (ed.) *Modern Trends in Forensic Medicine – 3*. (London: Butterworths)
24. Needham, A. E. (1952). *Regeneration and Wound Healing*. (London: Methuen)
25. Prinsloo, I. and Gordon, I. (1951). Post-mortem dissection artefacts of the neck and their differentiation from ante mortem bruises. *S. Afr. Med. J.*, **25**, 358
26. Gonzales, T. A., Vance, M., Helpern, M. and Umberger, C. J. (1954). *Legal Medicine, Pathology and Toxicology*. (New York: Appleton–Century–Crofts)
27. Watson-Jones, R. (1952). *Fractures and Joint Injuries*, 4th Edn. (Edinburgh: E. and S. Livingstone)

Chapter 2

Regional Injury and Sequelae of Wounding

Gunshot wounds to the head, perforating stab wounds of the heart and lungs, fragmentation of the body by bomb blast, are all obviously immediately fatal events. In this chapter we are not concerned with immediate fatality but with the short and longer term effects of injury. Some of these, such as shock, occur in a few hours. Some, such as fat and thrombotic embolism may occur in a few days after injury, and some like neoplasia and fatal heart disease may be attributed to trauma after some years have elapsed.

Many cases of injury recover completely if the blood volume, pressure and flow are restored by appropriate treatment. Relatively few suffer delayed effects of the sort that we shall consider. In most cases the inflammatory response followed by the processes of repair exert beneficial healing effects. But even here the body's response can be deadly in certain situations. A notable example is the development of inflammatory oedema after brain injury. The relentless swelling of the cranial contents after cerebral contusion and laceration, if not controlled by steroid therapy, is one of the commonest causes of death after head injury.

It is convenient to consider the effects of wounding under three main headings though some of these categories may overlap. Some use the categories early, intermediate and late effects. This is a complex problem and other authors have approached it in different ways. Sevitt[1] considers the changes under the heads of local changes, regional injury, systemic reactions and complications.

The principal early or acute responses are tissue and organ injury with subsequent haemorrhage of varying degree and the acute inflammatory response. Death may occur at the early stage even before the inflammatory response has had time to become evident. In adult persons who die following severe injury, about one third are due to direct involvement of the brain, heart or kidney, either by the initial injury or because of pre-existing disease. Death in the remaining two thirds follows infection, respiratory and myocardial failure or bleeding from acute ulceration of the gut.

The causes of most acute deaths are usually obvious, involving massive injury to large blood vessels with subsequent bleeding. The effects of some forms of head injury and of blunt abdominal trauma are more subtle and require further elaboration here. Head trauma is very common and is often a major feature in accidents involving vehicles of various sorts. Abdominal injury is an increasingly common feature of children who have been injured non-accidentally and is also found in accidents in sport, in the home and at work.

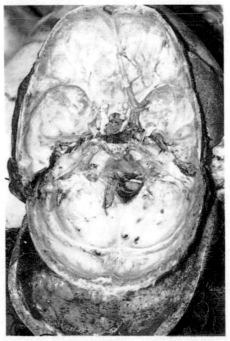

Figure 2.1 *Transverse fracture of the base of the skull through the middle cranial fossae and the sphenoid. This can follow a blow to the top of the head or to the front or back of the cranium*

29

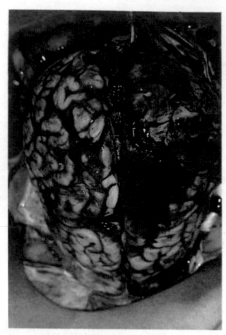

Figure 2.2 *Patches of blood on the top of the brain produced by tearing of a superficial dural vein*

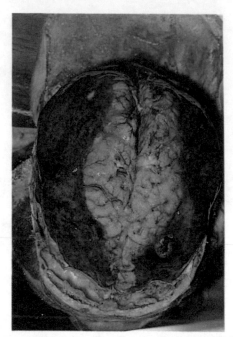

Figure 2.4 *Bilateral subdural haematomas of several months' duration*

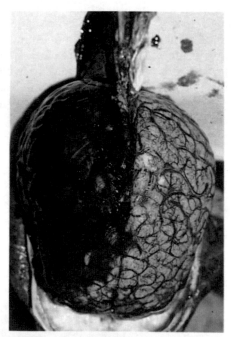

Figure 2.3 *Patches of blood on the top of the brain produced by tearing of a superficial dural vein*

CNS head injury

A blow to the head may produce a variety of effects which may occur singly or in combination. In order to understand and interpret the effects of head injury it is essential to have a detailed knowledge of the anatomy of the cranium and its contents. The skull can be regarded as a box with an oval section composed of a moderately elastic vault and a brittle perforated base. Thus a blow to the top of the head with a broad object

can sometimes lead to fissured fractures of the base of the skull running between the various cranial nerve foramina in the base (Figure 2.1). The brain itself lies relatively loosely in the skull anchored by the spinal cord and cranial nerves on in its underside, and by many small veins that run from the dura to the cranium (Figures 2.2, 2.3). Thus if the head is hit, the brain may move within the head relatively to the skull with the resultant tearing of vessels (Figure 2.4). This in turn leads to a slow collection of blood underneath the dura mater, a so-called subdural haematoma. Such haemorrhage is often associated with bleeding beneath the arachnoid mater so that clinical features may develop fairly rapidly. On the other hand, a pure subdural bleed may occur which may persist for years without any effect. The blood clot gradually breaks down and becomes encased in thick fibrous tissue (Figure 2.4). Such a lesion may follow a trivial rotational injury to the head, particularly in elderly people and, apart from adding a little to their usual state of confusion, may produce no other effect. However, such blood cysts, as they are sometimes called, may enlarge progressively by the imbibition of water caused by the increased osmolarity of the degenerating contents of the cyst. Progressive symptoms and signs of raised intracranial pressure may then appear weeks or months after the initial injury. Small repeated subsequent haemorrhages may lead to gradual enlargement of the haematoma.

Trauma to the head may therefore result in injury at the site of impact and injuries elsewhere to the brain which are often due to rotational movement of the brain within the skull. Injuries to the brain diametrically opposite to the point of impact are called contrecoup injuries.

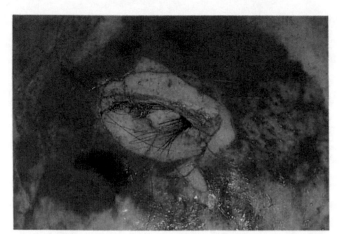

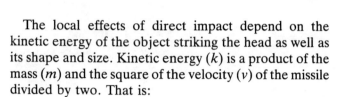

Figure 2.5 *Depressed fracture of the skull with pieces of bone and hair driven inwards with the fracture*

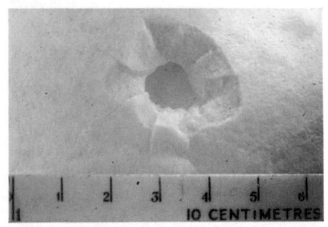

Figure 2.6 *View of the inside of a skull showing a small hole in the outer table and a larger one in the inner table*

The local effects of direct impact depend on the kinetic energy of the object striking the head as well as its shape and size. Kinetic energy (k) is a product of the mass (m) and the square of the velocity (v) of the missile divided by two. That is:

$$k = \tfrac{1}{2}mv^2$$

The effects of a hammer blow to the head derive largely from the mass of the hammer head, whereas the effects of a bullet arise largely from its velocity. Hammer blows produce a curved laceration in the scalp and a curved fracture in the skull at the first point of contact of the head of the hammer. The curvature of the injury clearly reflects the shape of the weapon. The skull is fractured and depressed inwards at this point and pieces of bone and hair may be driven into the cranial cavity (Figure 2.5). The hole in the outer table of the skull is smaller than that in the inner table as often occurs with low velocity blunt injuries to the head (Figure 2.6). Away from the point of impact the skull may show fissured fractures radiating away from the impact point.

If the head is struck with a broad object such as a plank, the point of impact is less clearly defined. Fracture lines may radiate in various directions in the vault and sides of the skull and may spread into the base as well. These fracture lines tend to follow the weaker parts of the base of the skull running through the cranial nerve foramina. The more solid buttresses of bone in the frontal and occipital parts and the transverse ridge of the petrous bones tend to resist the injury. Other common patterns of injury to the skull base are a transverse fracture anterior to the petrous bones running through the pituitary fossa. This often follows a blow to the frontal or occipital regions and is a frequent injury in road traffic accidents (Figure 2.1). Another pattern is the ring fracture: this runs around the foramen magnum and may follow a blunt injury to the vault of the skull. Equally, ring fractures of the occiput may follow injuries when the vertebral column tends to be forced upwards into the skull. This may occur when the

body falls a distance and lands on its feet. For example, walking on an asbestos roof causes the roof to collapse. Asbestos roofing is often used for farm buildings and out-buildings and falls of this sort form one of the lethal injuries that may occur in agricultural workers. Explosions of mines at sea likewise may cause ring fractures of the skull base or crush fractures of the vertebral bodies as the force of the explosion is transmitted from the deck of the ship through the feet and legs to the spine. It was not surprising that injuries of this sort were found in the crews of mine-sweeping craft in the last World War and in parachutists.

Ring fracture of the occiput may involve the vertebral artery as it enters the cranium. Thus will lead to intense pressure on the hind brain by extradural haemorrhage from the torn artery. This particular arterial injury is often difficult to detect at autopsy and is shown best by injecting radio-opaque material into the vertebral vessels low in the neck where they enter the vertebral canal, and then taking a radiograph of the skull and cranial region before the brain is removed.

Vascular injuries of various sorts are a frequent accompaniment of head injury and practically any blood vessel of any size may be involved. We have already discussed injuries to the vertebral arteries. However, the middle meningeal artery and its branches are involved much more frequently when there is head injury. The vessel may be involved either directly by a fracture of the skull where the artery lies, or indirectly following blows to the jaws and face exerting distracting forces on the vessel. We shall say more of the mechanisms of such injuries in the chapter on injuries that may occur in sporting accidents (Chapter 5).

The main middle meningeal artery is usually involved; its posterior division is affected less frequently. The result of tearing of this vessel is the formation of a haematoma outside the dura at the site of arterial damage. This is an extradural haemorrhage and may accumulate quickly resulting in compression of the

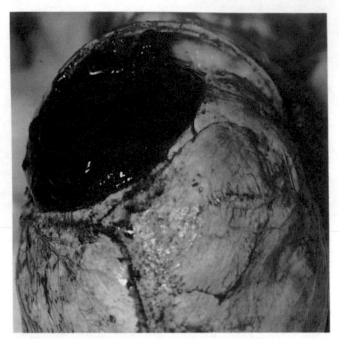

Figure 2.7 *Extradural blood clot due to rupture of the middle meningeal artery following skull fracture*

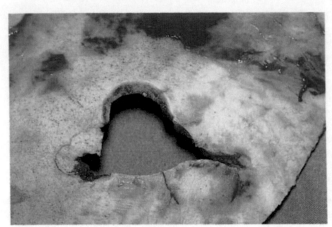

Figure 2.8 *Axe wound of skull showing bevelling at the top at the point of impact and splintering of the lower fragment. A typical chop wound*

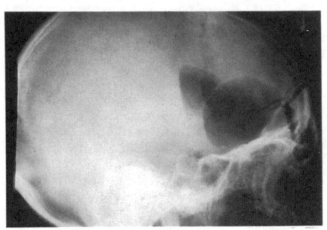

Figure 2.9 *Intracranial air from a frontal bone fracture involving the frontal sinus. (Courtesy of Dr T. D. Hawkins)*

brain and coma (Figure 2.7). However, in about two-thirds of the cases there is a latent interval of several hours duration. Extra dural haemorrhage is an eminently curable neurosurgical condition and early recognition of its possible occurrence is important. The diagnosis is often confused by other factors such as drunkenness. Careful examination of head wounds before they are sutured may be of considerable value in diagnosis. This is well illustrated by the death of a young man admitted to an Accident Department with a head wound said to have been caused by a fall against a door post. Both he and his brother, who took him to hospital, were drunk. The head wound was thought to be a laceration, it was sutured and the man sent home. He died 4h later of an extradural haematoma caused by an axe wound to his head. At autopsy the wound was incised, not lacerated, and there was a chop-fracture in the skull that had severed the middle meningeal artery (Figure 2.8). Failure to recognize the axe wound was one of the errors in this case but any head wound in a confused person should be regarded with great circumspection. A radiograph of the skull is mandatory and the patient should preferably be observed in a hospital bed for at least 24h. It is also essential to obtain an expert radiological opinion of the skull X-rays. Hair-line fractures are easily missed by the tiro. Likewise, the presence of intracranial air from fractures through the nasal sinuses can easily be overlooked (Figure 2.9).

Traumatic haemorrhage is also found in the subarachnoid space. It is most often due to direct contusion of the cerebral gyri which show linear bruising along the crests of the gyri. Subarachnoid haemorrhage may also follow traumatic haemorrhage into the brain itself, the

blood then bursting through into the subarachnoid space (Figure 2.10). However, in general forensic practice most of the cases of fatal subarachnoid haemorrhage are caused by the rupture of small 'berry' aneurysms in the arteries of the circle of Willis. These usually occur on the anterior part of the circle and are more frequently seen in hypertensive subjects, particularly in those with coarctation of the aorta. The aneurysms occur at the sites of medial muscular deficiency, a form of arterial dysplasia, which is found in other animals as well as in man[2]. It is reasonable to assume that this common medial deficiency only produces effects when hypertension is coexistent. The aneurysms may rupture into the subarachnoid space, and often do so. However, they may also adhere to the inferior surface of the brain and rupture, in various directions into the brain itself. Atherosclerotic aneurysms of the basal arteries of the brain may also rupture and produce subarachnoid haemorrhage. In addition, abnormal bleeding states such as thrombocytopenia may lead to leakage of blood from otherwise normal vessels into the subarachnoid space.

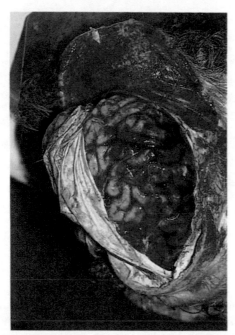

Figure 2.10   *Cerebral hemisphere with reflected dura showing subarachnoid haemorrhage rising up from the base of the brain*

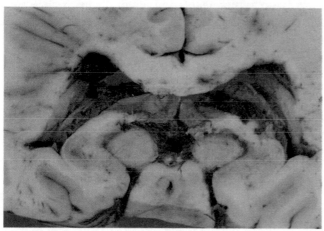

Figure 2.11   *Laceration and haemorrhage into the corpus callosum following rotational head injury*

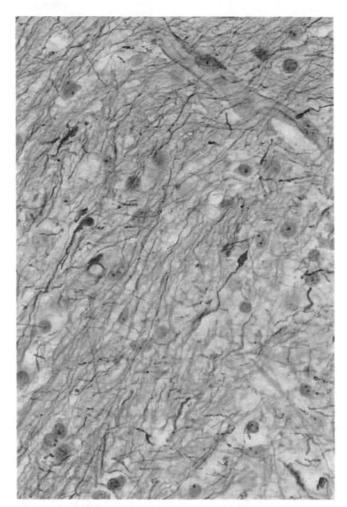

Figure 2.12   *Section of brain showing a fragmented nerve fibre with a 'retraction ball' at one end indicating diffuse neuronal injury*

Various sorts of trauma can cause subarachnoid bleeding. Contusion of the brain, as we have said already is one factor. Overdistension of thin-walled blood vessels may also be a factor as is seen in deaths from asphyxia where a combination of congestion and hypoxic damage to the vessel wall may lead to leakage of blood. Similar events occur in explosive blast injury.

Bleeding from small aneurysms into the brain tissue itself usually follows hypertensive or diabetic vascular diseases. Multiple small traumatic haemorrhages occur more commonly in head injury than is realized and it is the reaction to these multiple lesions that may lead to intractable cerebral oedema. They are caused by chafing of the surface of the brain on the inside of the skull and twisting of the brain, both of which occur in deceleration injuries. The haemorrhages often appear

as linear splits in the substance of the brain (Figure 2.11) and are frequent in the corpus callosum which is a fixed structure about which the cerebral hemispheres may attempt to rotate when the head is suddenly brought to a stop. Formalin fixation of the brain for 3 weeks followed by careful dissection is often the only way to show these lesions. Dissection of the fresh brain at autopsy is probably one of the reasons why these lesions are not more often recognized.

The term concussion is often used to imply a relatively minor but recoverable degree of brain damage following head injury. Recent work has, however, revealed that the borderline between concussion and cerebral contusion is by no means clear. Careful histological studies of the brains of concussed people have revealed a variety of neuronal changes[3]. However, because of the fact that concussed persons usually recover a lot of the work has been done in experimental animals.

A variety of changes has been described, such as fragmentation and chromatolysis of Nissl substance. In addition the axons may show twisting, fragmentation and swelling of the broken ends with accompanying demyelination (Figure 2.12). The problem in interpretation of these findings is to decide whether they are

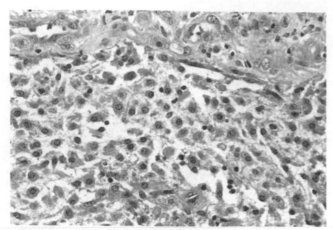

Figure 2.13 *Swollen vacuolated microglia (compound granular corpuscles) at the edge of an area of cerebral necrosis*

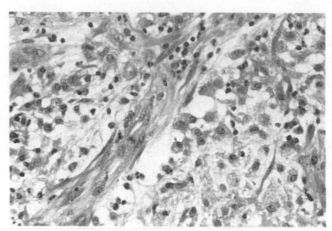

Figure 2.15 *Fibroblastic and glial reaction at the edge of necrotic brain tissue*

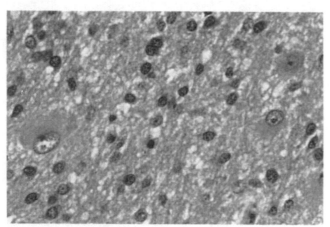

Figure 2.14 *Astroglial reaction to necrotic brain tissue*

primarily due to injury or are secondary to ischaemia, or pressure due to cerebral oedema. Such changes are often seen in the hind brain which is both readily susceptible to trauma by virtue of its surroundings and is also peculiarly liable to be affected by the coning effect of brain oedema.

Later histological changes consist of calcium and iron deposits at the sites of damaged neurons and balls of retraction which are clubbed ends of degenerate fragmented nerve fibres. There is also a brisk adjacent reaction of microglia which swell up and are deeply argyrophilic when stained by silver methods such as that of Weil–Davenport. These later changes are not specific for traumatic damage but are common sequelae of any form of neuronal injury.

The determination of the age of wounds in the central nervous system is based on essentially the same principles as those employed for the ageing of wounds elsewhere in the body. In the brain, however, there is a wider variety of reacting cells and it is also possible to sample and examine the cerebrospinal fluid that bathes the surface and cavities of the brain. The presence of fresh blood indicates recent injury. Haemolysis with staining of the supernatant occurs a few hours after

injury and fresh xanthochromia does not develop until 12–24 h have elapsed. Provided that there is not recurrent bleeding the yellow colour of the cerebrospinal fluid can be expected to fade in 2 weeks or so.

Within the brain tissue itself the oligodendrocyte is the first cell to react. In a few hours they swell and show cytoplasmic vacuolation. Later the microglia enter the region of tissue damage, being clearly evident at about 12 h after injury. These cells then phagocytose necrotic debris, swelling to form compound granular capsules (Figure 2.13). These are readily visible 24 h after injury. Haemosiderin appears, as at other sites in the body, in a few days and the macrophages migrate around adjacent blood vessels that become encrusted with iron. However, it must be remembered that ferruginization of capillaries and small arteries is a feature of many forms of brain damage and is not an unusual feature in the brains of the aged.

Astroglia are the last to respond to brain injury. The cells swell about the fourth day and collect around the area of tissue damage (Figure 2.14). By about 3 or 4 weeks the damaged area is replaced by a tangle of glial fibres and astrocytes. At about 8 weeks scarring is complete. Fibroblasts also play a part in this process, being derived from the adventitial sheath of adjacent arteries and from bits of dura that may have been driven into the area of damaged brain (Figure 2.15). Such a scar is often adherent to the brain membranes and may form a focus of abnormal electrical activity which may result in epilepsy.

At the end of the process when the damaged brain is represented by a haemosiderin-stained cyst with a glial wall or by a depressed scar, the early changes in fragmented neurons may still be found and indeed may persist for years.

Not all vascular injuries in the head and neck have an immediate effect. Some are delayed because the vessel, though damaged, may not be completely torn. The effect of this is to lead to the formation of an aneurysm which may burst on a much later occasion.

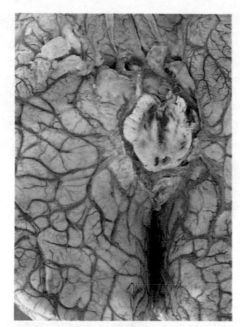

Figure 2.16 *Transverse section of pons showing linear haemorrhages due to venous rupture*

We shall discuss this matter in detail in relationship to delayed rupture of the traumatized thoracic aorta. In the neck vertebral artery aneurysms may arise from fracture dislocation or by manipulation of the neck or from severe osteophytic distortion of the cervical spine[4].

Weight, velocity and shape all contribute to the pattern of injury within the head. To these factors must also be added the rotational component of the brain within its dural membrane and bony case. On impact the brain twists and rebounds within the skull so that damage to parts of the brain directly opposite to the impact point frequently occurs. Several theories have been propounded to explain the occurrence of contrecoup injuries[5].

The struck hoop theory likens the skull on impact to a deformed hoop. The ovoid shape of the skull is exaggerated and the brain opposite to the point of impact collides with the deformed skull.

The theory of brain displacement was proposed by Russel. It postulates continued movement of the brain within the skull after the bony case has been brought to a halt.

Goggio postulates a change in pressure gradients within the brain. At the site of impact the intracerebral pressure is raised whereas in the opposite side the pressure is lowered, thus allowing a bursting effect in that area.

Finally, there is little doubt that rotational forces occur in either deceleration or acceleration and these can lead to contrecoup injury.

Most contrecoup injuries occur to the frontal, temporal and parietal parts of the brain. The occipital poles lying in the rounded capacious posterior fossa are less often involved. This suggests that impact of the frontal and temporal poles against the irregular floors and borders of the anterior and middle cranial fossae is an important factor in contrecoup damage.

Traumatic lesions of the brainstem and spinal cord may be part of the spectrum of injuries seen in road traffic accidents, in agricultural injuries, in civil strife and so on. The pathogenesis of the lesions is not always easily explained, particularly the central locations of the traumatic lesions in brainstem and cord.

Lesions of the brainstem in cases of fatal head injury may be primary or secondary. Secondary lesions are common and follow swelling of the injured brain leading to downward displacement of the pons and hind brain with compression against the clivus of the skull and borders of the foramen magnum. The effects of this are to impede the venous return with the formation of linear anteroposterior haemorrhages derived from anteroposterior ruptured veins (Figure 2.16). These may become confluent and lead to rapid death. In recent times it has been appreciated that arteriolar and capillary compression may also be an important factor in the genesis of secondary lesions of the brainstem. This is due to stretching and squeezing of the circumferential and perforating vessels of the hind brain as the brain swells[6]. Secondary lesions may develop early or late after head injury, depending on the rate of swelling of the cerebral hemispheres. It should always be anticipated as a sequel of brain injury and attempts to prevent it by the use of dexamethasone are a routine part of neurosurgical practice. Other parts of the brain may be rendered ischaemic by the pressure of swollen brain forcing other parts of it against rigid structures. The cingulate gyrus may be displaced under the falx cerebri and the midbrain may be forced against the tentorium cerebelli causing haemorrhage and necrosis in it. The compressed midbrain shows a notch on its lateral side called Kernohan's notch. The process explains how clinical signs may appear on the same side as that of the damaged cerebral hemisphere.

There are several sorts of primary brainstem lesions that are caused by injury. Local fractures of the basiocciput may be responsible for severe laceration of the brainstem. A blow to the back of the head may cause a contrecoup injury, the result being many midsagittal petechiae in the pons and tegmentum of the midbrain. Lateral displacement of the stem may follow injury to the side of the head; this causes the brainstem to impinge on the edge of the tentorium cerebelli. Displacement of the more mobile cerebral hemisphere may also lead to the lateral stretching of the brainstem with subsequent damage.

Cranial nerve lesions may be produced by stretching or by compression from swollen adjacent brain. The third and sixth nerves are most often involved, the former because of its proximity to a compressed swollen uncus and the latter because of its long tenuous intracranial course. Finally, the circulation of cerebrospinal fluid may be impeded by interruption of the basal foramina when the brain is displaced downwards. This occurs especially when the cerebellar tonsils herniate into the foramen magnum, a process known as coning.

Not all of the foci of ischaemic damage found in the brain following severe head injury may be due to trauma to the head itself. Fat embolism is a common accompaniment of trauma and though it often does not produce clinical effects it can lead to tiny foci of brain necrosis.

The extent of fat embolism within the brain can be slight but fatal if it occurs in the vessels of a vital area such as the brainstem. Furthermore, the degree of trauma to adipose tissue need not be great to produce this effect. A recent example in this department was the report of a woman who failed to regain consciousness after the extraction of a rear molar tooth and who died of fat embolism 10 hours later. The source of the embolic fat was a maxillary pad of fat damaged during the course of a difficult extraction. Histological examination of the brain revealed numerous fat emboli in vessels of the brainstem but few in those of the cerebral hemispheres.

Spinal cord injuries may assume a variety of forms, though the bulk of them are due to direct cord compression by a fracture dislocation of a vertebra. The injury can be severely crippling and though the number of cord injuries in most Western countries is no more than 20 per million of the population they provide desperate and complicated cases for the surgeon and physician. Not only is the initial treatment difficult but the management of the many sequelae demands great skills by doctor and nurse.

Less common causes of spinal cord injury are gunshot wounds and wounds from other flying missiles. Stab wounds, which are increasingly frequent as a mode of homicide, occasionally injure the spinal cord by chance.

Fracture dislocation of the spine usually involves the lower cervical and lower thoracic regions. The latter may be a feature of seat-belt injuries. The usual case is a violent flexion of the spine as may occur in a motor vehicle accident or following a fall from a height on to the feet. Amongst sports accidents fracture dislocation of the spine is most common amongst diving enthusiasts. Damage to the cord can also occur without fracture dislocation following hyperflexion. This may be due to previous narrowing of the spinal canal by osteoarthrosis which predisposes the flexed cord to ischaemic damage.

When the cord is examined at necropsy the lesion may consist of softening and haemorrhage into the central part, the damaged area being surrounded by normal cord. Furthermore, this area of necrosis and haemorrhage (haematomyelia) may gradually extend converting a paraplegia into a quadriplegia. This curious phenomenon may be explained by invoking damage to the blood supply to the cord. Key arteries from the vertebral and intercostal arteries contribute to the blood supply by the anterior spinal artery[7]. Damage to any of these vessels may explain extensive cord necrosis. Damage to these key vessels may incur extensive necro-

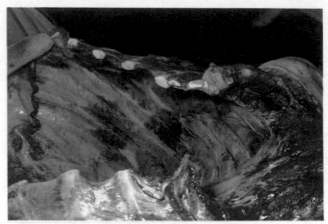

Figure 2.17 *Extensive pleural bruising over fractured ribs that have penetrated the pleura*

sis of the spinal cord in the thoracolumbar region and yet there is little or no vertebral injury. On the other hand, it is surprising how infrequently cord damage occurs in those who survive dissecting aneurysms of the thoracic aorta where the intercostal arteries are frequently involved at their origins.

Thoracic and abdominal injury

Other forms of regional injury involve the thorax and abdomen. Severe blunt injury to the chest is common and is responsible, in part, for about a quarter of the deaths of those involved in road traffic accidents. Injury to the chest wall is not so often associated with the devastating effects that are seen in head injury. Local injury may lead to bruising of the tissues of the chest wall and underlying lung which may produce only minor clinical effects. However, local chest injury, as may be caused by a blow with a fist or an object at work, is occasionally blamed for the occurrence or recrudescence of heart and lung disease. We shall discuss this matter later in the chapter.

The effects of generalized crushing injury depend not only upon the force of trauma but also on the age of the subject. A lorry wheel passed over the chest of a 10-year-old cyclist: the chest itself was little damaged and the elastic ribs were not broken. The cause of death was a small tear in a right inferior lobar branch of a pulmonary artery. The injury was caused by crushing of the lung by the pliable chest wall. In older people however, crush injury such as occurs in a car driver involved in a crash will involve rib and sternal fractures.

Sternal fractures usually follow a direct impact to the breast bone by an object such as the steering wheel of a car. If extensive, this fracture, coupled with fractured ribs, can form a serious impediment to breathing as the front of the chest moves inwards on inspiration, thus impairing the aeration of the lungs. This is the so-called flail chest. The sternum and vertebral column may also be broken by forced hyperflexion of the chest, as for example when a pedestrian is struck by a motor vehicle

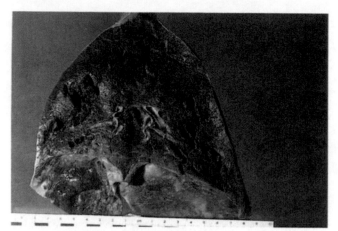

Figure 2.18 *Intrapulmonary haemorrhage into the lower lobe of the lung following crush injury without pleural penetration*

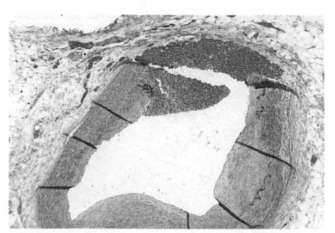

Figure 2.19 *Bruising of epicardial fat and rupture of the coronary artery*

from behind[1]. Several ribs may be broken by the same injury and again a flail chest may be the result.

Broken ribs of themselves are not necessarily a serious hazard, particularly if the parietal pleura is not broken by the fractured rib. It is quite common to find broken ribs with extensive parietal pleural bruising in victims of road traffic deaths, or for that matter in those in whom resuscitative attempts have been attempted and have failed. The pleura, though bruised, is intact (Figure 2.17). These fractures may be associated with fat and bone marrow embolism in the lungs but even this is not always of clinical consequence. Once the ribs are broken there may be varying degrees of bleeding into the pleural cavities. Such haemothoraces may be quite small or sometimes large enough to collapse the lung. Broken ribs may also penetrate the lung producing combinations of pneumothorax and haemothorax. Occasionally a pneumothorax may be advantageous under such circumstances in that the lung collapses and bleeding from it is reduced.

Puncture of the lung by broken ribs may also lead to intrapulmonary haemorrhage with consequent asphyxia. However, it must not be forgotten that asphyxiation by blood in road traffic victims is not always brought about by severe injury. Damage to the nose and mouth may cause considerable bleeding leading to asphyxia in a semi-conscious patient. The maintenance of a clear airway in survivors of such accidents is consequently an important aspect of the first-aid measures instituted at the scene. Extensive intrapulmonary haemorrhage can also occur without a break in the pleural surface of the lung. Central contusions of this sort may be extensive and are probably produced by squashing of the lung and its parabronchial vessels (Figure 2.18).

A good deal of alveolar rupture is due to the fact that the alveoli cannot empty quickly enough when the impact occurs. The alveoli over-distend and if emphysema is already present they may burst. Extensive alveolar rupture is a special feature of blunt injuries to the lung: this is often accompanied by generalized haemor-

rhage into the lung. It is probably due to the effects of blast pressure on the outer chest wall rather than being caused by a wave of pressure travelling down the trachea. We shall say more of this under civil strife (Chapter 7).

Compared to the lung the heart is relatively immune to blunt injury. It suffers most from compression injury following severe deceleration with consequent tearing of various cardiac structures (q.v.). Direct blunt injury may cause myocardial contusion with superficial bruising and laceration of cardiac muscle fibres. Occasionally the traumatized ventricle may rupture. This occurs most often with the thin right ventricle. Not only is the ventricle thin but it may also have a good deal of adipose tissue infiltration of its wall. Occasionally a ruptured right ventricle might ensue after chest compression during attempted resuscitation. This is particularly likely to happen if the pulmonary outflow tract is partly occluded by a large embolus.

Bruising may also occur on the anterior ventricular septum in the region of the left coronary artery (Figure 2.19). Injury to this region may lead to rupture of an atheromatous plaque with consequent exposure of plaque collagen leading to platelet aggregation and thrombosis. It is also possible to get thrombosis from traumatic endothelial injury in the absence of atheroma. This matter is clearly of great importance when the question of compensation may arise from the effects of cardiac ischaemia which might be attributed to work or other injury.

Subendocardial haemorrhage is a curious finding in many injured patients at necropsy. It usually takes the form of streaky haemorrhage beneath the endocardium of the ventricular septum and the left papillary muscles (Figure 2.20). It is seen in about 70% of those who died within 12 hours of road accident and in 40% of accident cases overall. The mechanism is obscure and it has sometimes been called a 'shock' lesion. Experimentally it can be produced by making animals hypotensive by bleeding. However, it is also seen in cases of severe

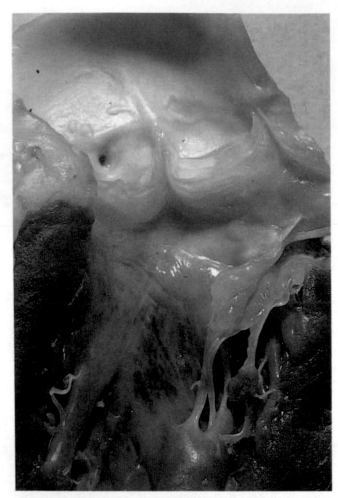

Figure 2.20 *Streaks of subendocardial haemorrhage on the ventricular septum in a person dying within a few hours of multiple injuries*

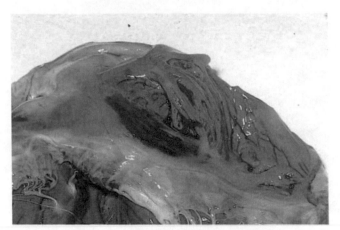

Figure 2.21 *Split in the wall of the right atrium due to deceleration injury*

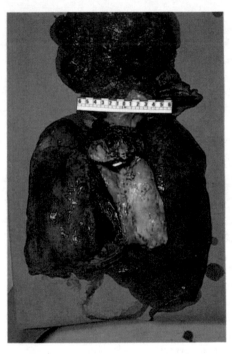

Figure 2.22 *Laceration of the aorta at the junction of the descending part of the arch and the thoracic portion. A common deceleration injury*

burns and in non-traumatic events such as bleeding into a cerebral tumour or some other acute intracranial event. A variety of mechanisms has been proposed, such as sympathetic overactivity, hypoxic dilatation of subendocardial capillaries that are ill-supported by the surrounding connective tissues, and so on. When examined microscopically the lesions are fresh consisting of intact erythrocytes, which suggests that the lesion was agonal.

The thoracic viscera, and in particular the heart and the aorta, are susceptible to deceleration injury, the lungs less so, unlike crushing injury when the reverse situation applies. Deceleration is caused by sudden arrest of the body at speed; mobile organs such as the heart by virtue of their mass continue to move forward and to tear themselves away at points of firm attachment to the thorax. The deceleration injuries may be relatively trivial or very severe, depending on the speed of the body at the moment of deceleration. At relatively slow speeds the deceleration injuries to the heart occur in its thinner posterior parts, common injuries being tearing of the pulmonary veins and inferior vena cava close to the points of cardiac entry. Often the lesions are only partial splits, the whole wall not being completely

transected. Tears in the atrial septum are frequently found anterior to the coronary sinus in the right atrium. Here again the split may be endocardial and not involve the full thickness of the atrial wall (Figure 2.21).

With more severe deceleration, tears in the veins and atrial septum may be complete, leading in the latter case to an acquired atrial septal defect. Similar tears can lead to ventricular septal defects but violent deceleration is often needed to produce this injury. Aircraft accidents produce severe deceleration injuries and in these accidents the heart and lungs may be found lying loose in the thorax or in the abdomen because the diaphragm ruptures as well.

The start of the descending thoracic aorta is another point where the heart is tethered to the posterior thoracic wall. Rupture of the aorta at this site is a common

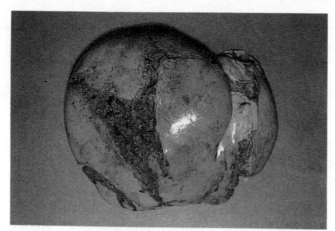

Figure 2.23 *Lacerations on the superior aspect of the liver following the contours of the coronary and triangular ligaments*

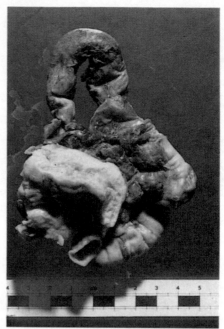

Figure 2.24 *An old fibrotic haematoma in the mesentery of a child injured non-accidentally*

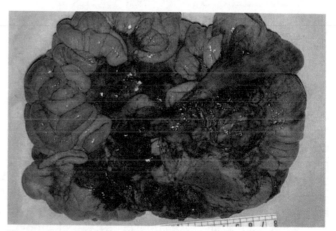

Figure 2.25 *Recent mesenteric bruising on a child injured by blows on the abdominal wall*

form of deceleration injury (Figure 2.22). The full thickness of the wall may not be breached and the adventitial coat of the aorta will prevent escape of blood from the vessel. Even if blood does escape a pleural or mediastinal haematoma may restrict leakage of blood into the thoracic cavity. This is clearly an important post-traumatic complication to recognize clinically. If a chest radiograph reveals broadening of the mediastinum in an accident victim further investigation and surgical treatment is imperative. Individuals may survive for 24 h or more after aortic rupture; the condition is readily curable surgically if thought about and recognized. About 85% of persons with thoracic aortic transection die at once. About 8% die whilst being transported for surgical treatment, but for the few who survive for operation the mortality is low – of the order of 5–20%. In 2% or so of all cases the diagnosis is overlooked and a healed aortic tear, or a calcified mediastinal haematoma may be discovered as a legacy of previous aortic damage. The usual site for traumatic aortic rupture is the descending part of the aortic arch. Occasionally, however, the vessel may rupture in the ascending part of the arch or at the level of the diaphragm. In elderly subjects the aorta which is calcified and atheromatous may fracture at the level of the diaphragm. This happened to an elderly cyclist on the perimeter of an airfield. He was tipped from behind by the wing of a taxi-ing plane, fell off his bicycle and broke his aorta at diaphragmatic level.

Abdominal injuries are the last regional group that we shall consider in this chapter. They can be caused by direct blows to the abdominal wall or by acute flexion injury, or by deceleration. As with deceleration injuries in the thorax, the same principles apply. The heavy organs continue to move forward when the body is arrested at speed and they tend to break loose at their points of attachment to the fixed posterior abdominal wall. For example, tears appear in the capsule of the liver near to the attachments of the coronary and triangular ligaments (Figure 2.23). The spleen and kidneys

tend to tear away from the vessels at their hila. Curiously enough, this is more likely to happen to the right kidney as compared to the left. The small intestine is a heavy mass of tissue and deceleration injuries tend to appear in the ileocaecal mesentery and in the mesenteric root. All of these injuries may produce a large haemoperitoneum or retroperitoneal haemorrhage in the paracolic gutters in the case of renal pedicular damage. It is surprising how often right renal pedicular haemorrhage is found at autopsy following a quite trivial fall, as for example following collapse from a heart attack. The right kidney is probably more mobile and less well supported than the left which may explain the discrepant findings of traumatic renal pedicular haemorrhage. Any injury that causes a sudden rise of intra-abdominal pressure will lead to diaphragmatic rupture.

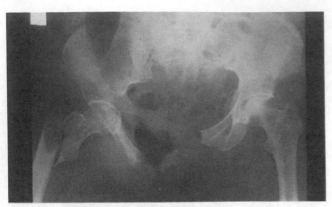

Figure 2.26 *Severe crush fracture of the pelvis with tearing of pelvic organs including the urethra*

A direct blow, violent deceleration, a severe jack-knife movement as follows falls on the feet, or constraint by a seat belt, may all cause diaphragmatic rupture. The paracentral left leaf of the diaphragm usually ruptures and the stomach, splenic flexure of the colon and the left lobe of the liver may enter the thorax through the hole. Severe hyperflexion may also cause liver rupture, explosive overdistension of the gut which bursts – usually the anterior colon or small bowel is involved – and crushed fracture of the thoracolumbar spine may also result.

Direct blows to the abdominal wall are an increasingly common cause of injury and death. These may occur in vehicular, sporting or industrial accidents but are of particular importance in children who have been injured non-accidentally. Repeated blows to the abdominal wall cause large mesenteric haematomas (Figures 2.24, 2.25), splits in the liver that may heal, and rupture of spleen and kidney if the blow is more posterior. Of all the abdominal organs the pancreas is least vulnerable to injury because of its deep-lying posterior position. However, in recent times the incidence of injury has risen from 1% to 10% in all cases of abdominal trauma. It is usually damaged by localized injury such as a steering wheel, ill-fitting seat belt, or by a direct blow. The classical mid-line injury splits the pancreas in two and the duct ruptures leaking secretions around. Usually, however, adjacent organs such as spleen, liver, bowel and kidney are often involved and the pancreatic injury may be overlooked. The result is that pancreatic enzymes continue to leak into the tissues and pancreatitis, sepsis, secondary haemorrhage and fistulas may prove lethal[8].

Other viscera may rupture when traumatized and are particularly liable to do so when distended. For example, the stomach may burst on injury, after a large meal, or when a good deal of air and water distends the viscus, as may occur in drowning. Rupture of the bladder may also occur when it is distended and traumatized. The viscus usually gives way in the dome and it is not surprising that this phenomenon is seen in alcoholics from time to time. Far and away the commonest cause

of rupture of the bladder and membranous urethra, however, is a crush fracture of the bony pelvis (Figure 2.26).

Sequelae of injury

It is convenient to consider the latent effects of trauma under two heads, though some overlap occurs between the two groups. The local effects sometimes relate directly to the organ itself, for example, the effects that may ensue from a traumatic thrombosis of the left coronary artery, or they may relate to structures served by the damaged organ. For example, damage to the spinal cord creates a chain of problems in the urinary tract caused by stasis of urine.

The general effects tend to be manifest throughout the body and the most common, controversial and least understood is shock. Other general manifestations include emboli of thrombi, fat or air, septicaemia from infected wounds, renal failure, pneumonia and various manifestations of stress such as acute gastrointestinal ulceration.

It is a tragic fact that the majority of people who sustain severe head injuries die shortly after the accident. The vast majority of these people are victims of road traffic accidents when consumption of alcohol is an important adjuvant factor. In a recent series 41% died within a few hours of admission to hospital, 34% survived less than a week, 13% less than a month and only 12% survived one or more months[9]. The survivors of severe head injury present considerable problems in nursing and other management. They often fall into the category of young, chronic disabled, but are often demented. Some are hyperphagic, presumably because of hypothalmic injury and become very heavy and difficult to move. Others are violent and aggressive. Such cases, though small in number, are a serious problem for all neurosurgical units. A few of the young survivors become akinetic mutes and may survive for many years. They usually have sustained head injury without skull fracture and were initially decerebrate after the injury. We have seen such cases in Cambridge: one survived for 3 years to die of terminal respiratory infection. The initial causative event was probably a severe distortion of the brain with considerable shearing of structures within the brain substance. At post-mortem examination there is often little that is obvious to the naked eye. There may be scattered small areas of sunken cortical damage with haemosiderin staining of the lesions and of the adjacent meninges, particularly in the areas of contrecoup, such as the frontal and temporal poles. Similar small lesions are scattered throughout the brain around the aqueduct, in the superior cerebellar peduncles and in the corpus callosum. Histological examination reveals widespread degeneration of nerve fibres, as previously described. It is often not possible to find focal lesions to explain the Wallerian type degeneration of the fibres and the assumption is that they are caused by widespread shearing of the brain on deceleration[10].

The question of a relationship between trauma and the genesis of neoplasms is a vexed one. So far as the brain is concerned there is little evidence for this. However, Cushing and Eisenhardt[11] reviewing 313 patients with meningioma found a history of trauma to the head in 101.

Perhaps the most telling case was that of a newborn child with a skull fracture due to forceps delivery who subsequently developed a meningioma in the injured falx.

The pituitary gland is often found to be involved in fatal head injuries. Haemorrhages and necrosis are found equally in the anterior and posterior lobes. Transection of the pituitary stalk is a frequent event and haemorrhage into the pituitary capsule is common due to tearing of small peripheral adjacent vessels. These phenomena are all found in fatal cases. Yet it is surprising how rarely pituitary dysfunction follows head injury. Only about 0.1% of closed head injuries who recover show any signs of pituitary deficiency. The cranial nerves are other extrusions from the brain that may be damaged. The manifestation may be early or late. The early lesions are due to stretching or tearing of the nerves at the time of injury. The late effects may be due to the involvement of the nerves in organized blood clot or are caused by the effects of continually raised intracranial pressure.

About 3% of those who survive head injury show cranial nerve palsies affecting the third, fourth and sixth nerves. Other nerves such as the fifth and seventh may be involved if a fracture involves the nerve foramina. Defects of smell due to olfactory nerve damage are not infrequent following fractures of the frontal and ethmoid bones. Blindness may ensue if the optic nerves or chiasma are torn. Transient cortical blindness is probably due to trauma to the calcarine areas of the occipital poles and has a good prognosis. It is probably due to bruising and oedema of the occipital poles which subsequently subsides.

Long-term results of spinal cord injury are many and varied. These are direct neural effects caused by loss of nerve supply to various organs. Paraplegia and quadriplegia are obvious examples as are difficulties in emptying the bladder and failure of ejaculation. More subtle are orthostatic hypertension and failure to adjust body temperature. Orthostatic hypertension which causes spells of syncope and light-headedness is probably due to a loss of peripheral sympathetic vascular tone and a reduced tissue turgor in the paralysed parts which allows fluid to collect there. It is especially seen in quadriplegic subjects. Failure to maintain body temperature is seen with cord lesions above the level of T8 and though not fully understood is partly explained by the inability of shivering to occur below the level of the lesion. Lack of shivering fails to compensate for heat loss.

The neurogenic bladder with its static pool of urine

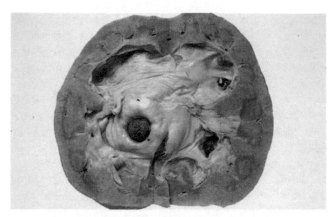

Figure 2.27 *Renal calculi from a paraplegic subject showing dilated renal pelvis and impacted stones in the pelvi-ureteric junction*

is a likely seat of infection in the paraplegic subject. Catheterization may be needed to keep the bladder empty and patients are taught to do this themselves following a rigid aseptic technique. Bladder infections can occur easily in these subjects and infection may ascend to the kidney with consequent inflammation and stone formation (Figure 2.27). Stones may also occur in the bladder itself and less often in the prostatic ducts and seminal vesicles. Inflammatory debris and bacteria provide a nidus upon which urinary salts are precipitated to form stones.

Immobility associated with spinal cord injury leads to ischaemic necrosis of skin at pressure points. This ulceration is initially due to the impedance of venous return leading to venous stasis and reduction of arterial inflow into the tissues. Venous stasis also promotes venous thrombosis and consequent pulmonary embolism. Venographic studies of paraplegic patients have revealed venous thrombi in the legs of the order of 58%. Another curious phenomenon is the formation of ectopic bone. This is the so-called paraosteoarthropathy of spinal cord injury. New bone is deposited alongside the hip, knee, shoulder and elbow joints. The mechanism is obscure, though a hypoxic factor is probably involved. The process is usually an incidental radiological finding but occasionally may be so exuberant as to limit the movement of the joint.

Further sequelae are consequent upon the complications. For example, hypertension is common in paraplegics secondary to the renal damage and amyloid disease may follow long-standing bed sores and chronic renal suppuration. The relationship of long-standing bladder infections in these patients to the incidence of bladder cancer is not proven.

We have already mentioned some of the sequelae of thoracic and abdominal injury. Perhaps one of the most vexed questions is the relationship of heart disease to previous trauma. The problem usually arises as a matter for compensation some years after the injury occurred. Direct trauma to the heart from a crushed sternum or broken ribs may lead to coronary artery damage with either atheromatous plaque rupture or endothelial damage leading to coronary thrombosis. More difficult to prove is the indirect effect of a severe injury of the heart. At the time of injury a variety of factors may operate to promote platelet aggregation with subsequent thrombus formation. Hypotension due to blood loss affects coronary flow and hypercoagulability following tissue injury are both thrombogenic factors. Fear and anxiety lead to catecholamine release which not only increases cardiac output but also predisposes again to platelet aggregation. Multiple platelet aggregates can cause sudden death in man[12] and have been produced experimentally by the infusion of ADP into the coronary arteries of pigs, when death again occurs. If coronary artery disease is already present the situation is clearly more fraught with danger. Disorders of rhythm and electrocardiographic changes are often associated with head injury; this may be related to muscle fibre damage or to subendocardial haemorrhage in the region of the conducting tissues. These changes may also impose an extra work load on the myocardium at the time of injury and may result in long-term myocardial damage from transient ischaemia due to variable coronary filling.

It is difficult to attribute to a previous injury some years before a causative role in heart disease. If the presence of hypotension, hypercoagulability and so on can be established at the time of injury the case is a more solid one but is still debatable. The sequelae of other thoracic and abdominal injuries and injuries to other organs will be dealt with elsewhere in this book. The rest of this chapter will be concerned with systemic responses to injury, in particular shock and embolism.

Of all the concepts in medicine, that of shock is the most difficult to define. Some regard it as a single entity characterized by a disturbance in volume, flow and distribution of various body fluids. Others subdivide it into traumatic, cardiogenic, septic and anaphylactic shock[13]. In this section we shall regard shock basically as a state of affairs leading to a reduction of capillary blood flow leading to cellular damage in many tissues and organs. The extent of the damage varies from tissue to tissue depending on supply and demand and the accumulation of waste products which are removed at varying rates. As shock develops the condition gets more complex as organs fail at different rates and the interdependence of one organ upon another varies from time to time.

Crush injuries are often associated with severe shock culminating in renal failure and dangerous hyperkalaemia from the damaged tissues. The clinical management of these cases is complex and there is a tendency to single out one particular feature of the shock syndrome and to concentrate on that. For example, the Moorgate Underground Tube Disaster involved many crush injuries. Two of these were trapped for several hours and developed the so-called crush syndrome consisting of oligaemia, hyperkalaemia and haematuria.

Treatment of the condition by aggressive fluid therapy and the judicious use of diuretics can often save them, but designations of this sort and others such as shock lung, fat embolism and so on, ignore the complex interconnections of many damaged organs in the shocking process[14].

A reduced cardiac output is a later feature which is common to most of the varieties of shock that have been described and when the shock is due to haemorrhage the peripheral vascular resistance is increased. However, this is not always the case. In traumatic shock alone there is an initial hyperdynamic state with an increased cardiac output and reduced vascular resistance occurring early on after the injury before and during the time of maximal hypotension. Sepsis will also give rise to shock characterized by a reduced peripheral resistance and increased cardiac output.

Initially then the striking physiological response to each of the various types of agents causing shock is an attempt to increase cardiorespiratory function. This arises from the effects of stress on the brainstem cardiac centres generally increasing autonomic activity and from the effects of the breakdown products of cells such as vasoactive peptides, endotoxins and the like. This resultant increase of heart rate, myocardial contractility and alveolar ventilation leads to an increased cardiac output unless there is myocardial damage or a reduced blood volume. The blood volume is maintained by fluid drawn from the intercellular spaces and ultimately from the cells themselves. Many of the biochemical abnormalities of the shock syndrome are explained by this fluid shift.

At the same time as the various shifts of fluid are occurring a variety of haemostatic mechanisms are being activated either by the trauma, hypoxia or infection. The release of tissue thromboplastins from traumatized or hypoxic endothelial cells precipitates the important syndrome of disseminated intravascular coagulation (DIC). This consumption of platelets and coagulation factors may lead paradoxically to haemorrhage from wounds or drainage sites and into the skin as purpura. On the other hand, deposits of microthrombi in renal vessels may impair renal function and lead to cortical necrosis and in the brain they cause neurological symptoms and signs. In the lung the microthrombi may cause obstruction to the circulation and the presence of platelets in the pulmonary vessels leads to vascular spasm. Whether this is sufficient to explain the changes of the adult respiratory distress syndrome or shock lung, as it is sometimes called, is debatable.

The syndrome of acute respiratory insufficiency after surgery, major trauma or haemorrhage is a modern disease produced by the advent of successful methods of resuscitation from shock and trauma that was hitherto fatal. Many other conditions such as oxygen toxicity, fat embolism, drug overdose and so on can be associated with shock lung so it must be regarded as a non-specific pulmonary response[15]. The condition usually follows

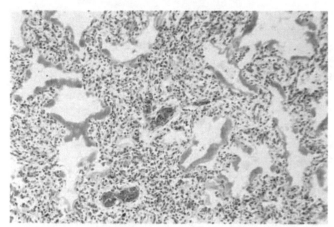

Figure 2.28 *Section of lung from a shocked patient maintained on a respirator, showing red hyaline membranes lining alveoli*

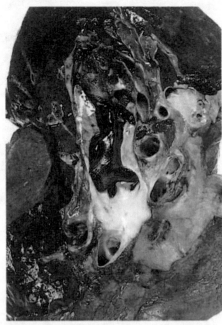

Figure 2.29 *Thrombus in the main pulmonary artery. The pink part is the original embolus; the deep red part is the red tail of the thrombus*

hours or days after an initial injury and is characterized in its later stages by progressive pulmonary insufficiency with hypoxia and hypercarbia leading finally to hypoxic cardiac arrest.

The pathological features in the lungs are greatly increased weight due largely to interstitial oedema with pulmonary fibrosis, the latter depending on the length or duration of the illness. The earliest stage seems to be interstitial oedema around larger blood vessels which gradually permeates the lung, finally getting into the alveolar walls. The lung vessels are dilated and there may be interstitial haemorrhages from these. Microthrombi may be seen in many blood vessels and there are often hyaline membranes in the alveoli. These are derived from desquamated alevolar lining cells and exudation of oedema fluid (Figure 2.28). In the final stage there is active proliferation of alveolar and interstitial cells. The latter appear so active as to give a pseudosarcomatous appearance. It has been postulated that a growth factor in the oedema fluid is responsible. This may be derived from platelets. The development of interstitial fibrosis often marks a point of no return when the lung is irretrievably damaged.

Bacteraemic and endotoxic shock may occur under a wide variety of conditions[16]; so far as this book is concerned it can be a complication of burns and road traffic accidents and in those maintained for any length of time in intensive care units. It is a serious condition with a mortality of more than 50%. It is caused by the liberation of toxins from a wide range of microbes, such as bacteria, fungi and viruses. The liberated toxins produce their effects by increasing capillary permeability and by causing widespread arteriolar and capillary thrombosis (DIC). In the later phase there may be myocardial damage as well and the resultant impairment of cardiac output is likely to prove fatal. Gram-negative bacteria are a common cause of endotoxic shock and it is important to realize that the use of antibiotics may liberate endotoxins from the organisms. The toxic end of the endotoxic molecule is lipid-A and

so the use of antibiotics has converted a septicaemia into an endotoxaemia.

Post-traumatic embolism is a common sequel of trauma. Emboli may consist of thrombi, fat, air or even particles of damaged tissue, such as bone marrow and traumatized liver. Trauma to any adipose tissue such as bone marrow or subcutaneous fat gives rise to fat emboli in the lungs. This is a frequent phenomenon and is usually not clinically apparent. Small thrombotic emboli derived from areas of tissue damage are also commonly found at necropsy in the lungs of traumatized people, again not having produced any clinical effects in life. The syndrome of massive pulmonary embolism is well documented. The episode occurs a week or so after injury and at autopsy a large coiled thrombus is found in the main pulmonary artery and its branches (Figure 2.29). The thrombus shows the characteristic features of formation ante-mortem. Its shape and branches conform to those of vessels such as the femoral or iliac veins and the surface is delicately ribbed with lines of Zahn caused by the layered components of thrombus. The layering is caused by sequential deposition of platelets and fibrin which then entangle erythrocytes, and so on. Undetached thrombi may be found in contralateral veins but quite often no thrombus can be found in the legs because it has all become detached to form the embolus. The finding of multiple thrombi in calf veins is difficult to interpret (Figure 2.30). It is a frequent finding at autopsy in patients who have been confined to bed for some time and yet show no evidence of pulmonary embolism.

It has been postulated that the cause of pulmonary embolism after trauma is an increased coagulability of

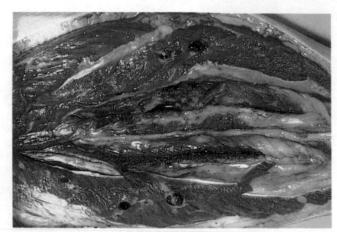

Figure 2.30 *Multiple thrombi in veins shown by incising calf muscles*

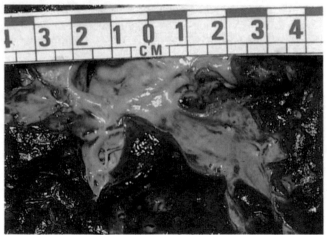

Figure 2.31 *A web of organized thrombus in a main branch of the pulmonary artery*

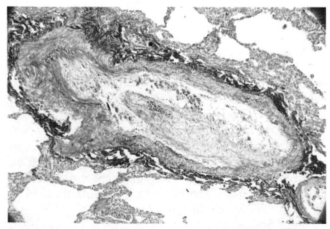

Figure 2.32 *Microscopically the web of organised thrombus consists of a strand of collagen (stained pink) crossing the vascular lumen*

the blood which is maximal about a week after injury. The hypercoagulable state is defined in terms of increased platelet adherence to glass bulbs when platelet-rich plasma from the patient is rotated within them. If, however, other tests for platelet stickiness are employed, such as exposing platelet-rich plasma to a bed of glass beads, increased stickiness can be observed at a few days after injury. This casts doubt on the significance of *in vitro* tests of platelet function as reflectors of the state of affairs in life. Platelet aggregation is, however, of undoubted importance in thrombus formation, particularly in the systemic arteries such as the coronaries. In veins, factors such as sluggish flow and endothelial trauma are potent factors in thrombogenesis. The effect of pulmonary embolism is to cause obstruction to the pulmonary circulation. This is partly due to the mass of the thrombus but is contributed to by spasm induced in the pulmonary artery and its branches when the embolus impacts. If the patient survives the embolus may become adherent to the artery wall and organizes ultimately to form a characteristic web of collagen on the intima (Figures 2.31, 2.32). Repeated emboli lead to progressive pulmonary hypertension, right ventricular hypertrophy and finally failure of the right ventricle (cor pulmonale).

Thrombotic emboli may come from a number of sources other than the legs, such as prostatic and uterine veins and indeed from any veins where adjacent tissue has been damaged. For example, fatal pulmonary embolism may follow axillary vein thrombosis after fracture of the arm.

Fat embolism is usually caused by bony injury and some say that evidence of it can be found in all cases. Trauma liberates fat from the marrow which enters the haversian systems and the venous circulation. The bones of children contain little fat so that fat embolism is less often seen in them. The second main cause of fat embolism derives from damaged subcutaneous tissue, either by burning or by trauma. A frequent cause of fat is the introduction of various metal prostheses into bones in orthopaedic operations. Replacement of the femoral head by a metal prosthesis is one of the common causes of fat embolism which may prove fatal[17] (Figures 2.33, 2.34). An increasingly common cause of pulmonary and cerebral fat embolism is the use of closed-chest cardiac massage. Jackson and Greendyke[18] found pulmonary fat emboli in 81% of such patients. The emboli were seen in alveolar capillaries and in larger vessels as well (Figure 2.35). Furthermore, rib fractures are not a prerequisite for the finding of fat embolism. The mere bending of the ribs may cause microfractures in the cancellous bones of the ribs and the pumping action of cardiac massage forces fat into the circulation. Much of this fat embolism is probably of little importance from the clinical point of view[19]. However, the finding of cerebral fat embolism at autopsy on such people cannot be ignored. The occasional report of mental impairment in persons recovered from cardiac

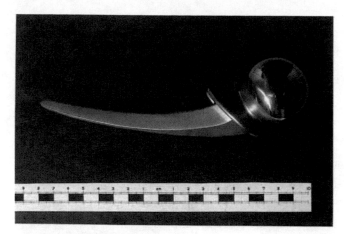

Figure 2.33 *A metal prosthesis used to replace the femoral head. The tapered end is inserted into the marrow cavity and is secured by cement*

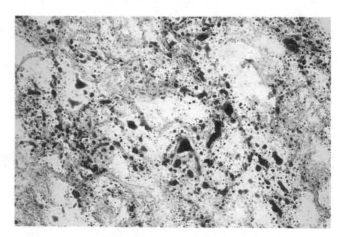

Figure 2.35 *Frozen section of lung stained by Oil Red O to show globules of fat in pulmonary capillaries and other vessels*

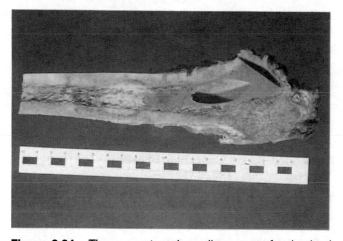

Figure 2.34 *The cement and a yellow area of pulverized necrotic fat providing a source for fat embolism*

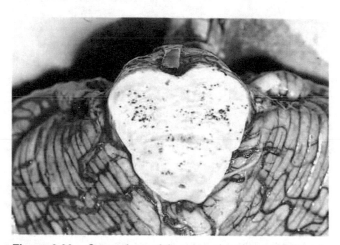

Figure 2.36 *Cut surface of the pons showing multiple petechial haemorrhages due to fat embolism*

massage coupled with the risks of cardiac contusion, splenic and hepatic rupture should occasion some thought as to the value of closed-chest massage in resuscitation.

The precise cause of the syndrome of fat embolism is still debated. The clinical effects seem to depend not so much on the volume of fat entering the pulmonary circulation but upon the speed with which it occurs. Zenker first described fat droplets in lung capillaries in 1862 and Wagner described the syndrome of fat embolism in 1865. The original view was that plugging of pulmonary capillaries by fat was the sole responsible factor. However, fat appears in lung capillaries in diabetic coma, phosphorus and carbon tetrachloride poisoning, and so on. From this derived the view that cerebral fat embolism must be shown before the syndrome can be diagnosed (Figure 2.36). Fat reaches the cerebral circulation via the foramen ovale, found in 25% of people at autopsy, or via bronchopulmonary anastomoses.

Another view is that the presence of fat causes red cell sludging and the formation of hyaline micro-

thrombi which contribute largely to the vascular obstruction. The third notion is that release of free fatty acids gives rise to a chemical pneumonitis and systemic effects[20].

Fat embolism usually occurs a few days after trauma though death may occur at once, as for example when a metal prosthesis is inserted into a bone. The full blown syndrome consists of dyspnoea with the appearance of fat in the sputum. As the fat enters the systemic circulation it may lead to pyrexia, cutaneous petechiae and cerebral signs. Later fat may appear in the urine and a few cases die of renal failure from extensive obstruction of glomerular capillaries.

Air embolism is a feature of any injury or procedure where a large vein is opened and air can get in because of the negative pressure within it; wounds of the neck and penetrating wounds of the lung can lead to pulmonary and systemic air embolism respectively (Figures 2.37, 2.38). In ordinary hospital practice surgery on the head and neck and the insufflation of air for diagnostic and therapeutic purposes, e.g. pneumoperitoneum or pneumothorax, can be followed by air embolism. The

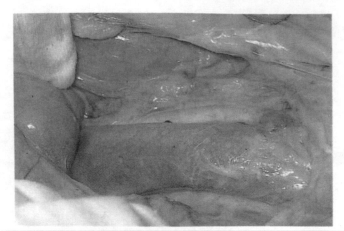

Figure 2.37 *Inferior vena cava full of air bubbles before it has been cut*

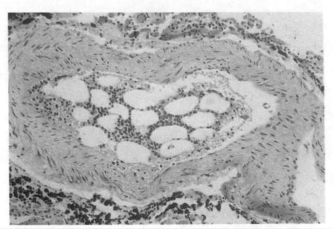

Figure 2.39 *Lung artery showing fatty bone marrow. This is bone marrow embolism following cardiac massage*

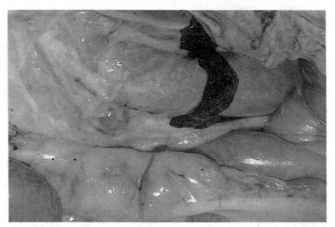

Figure 2.38 *The same inferior vena cava after it has been cut. This is the way to find venous air embolism at autopsy avoiding opening of large veins beforehand*

recent advent of open heart surgery has provided another way in which air can gain access to the circulation. The capacious veins of the gravid uterus are another potential portal for air following attempted abortion by insufflation. No reliable figures are available for the amount of air needed to cause the syndrome. Death has occurred following the insufflation of 300 ml of air into the vagina. Considerably less air is needed to prove fatal if it gains access to the coronary arteries as in cardiac surgery.

Fat and air embolism are not infrequently associated. This is particularly well illustrated by decompression sickness. In this condition individuals have been working under increased atmospheric pressure and have then been decompressed. If decompression occurs too rapidly nitrogen gas bubbles out of the tissues into the circulation. Nitrogen under pressure is mainly dissolved in fat and as the bubbles of gas emerge on decompression they fragment the adipose tissue cells leading to fat embolism as well. There is a good deal of fat in the marrow of long bones and vertebrae and the effect of emergent gas bubbles is to block capillary vessels in this tissue leading to areas of infarction of fatty marrow

and cancellous bone. Bone infarcts are a frequent sequela of decompression sickness. They are not exclusive to this disease: any condition leading to microvascular luminal occlusion, such as sickle-cell disease or microvascular compression as in Gaucher's disease can lead to bone infarction.

When Ericksen reviewed the literature on venous air embolism in 1844 he concluded that the effects were due to a primary arrest of the pulmonary circulation due to an air block and even as late as 1965 it was concluded that the mechanism was an obstruction of pulmonary capillaries by air bubbles. However, in 1968 Hartveit and her colleagues showed that the primary obstruction was due to fibrin plugs formed by the whipping up of bloody froth in the right ventricle. Fat droplets were also found mingled with the fibrin. It was concluded that these derived from coalescence of chylomicrons[21].

From the previous discussion it is clear that any foreign particle in the bloodstream is likely to generate microthrombi and droplets of fat, and the unravelling of the pathogenetic mechanisms in air, fat and other embolisms is by no means simple.

Tissue embolism is a well-recognized phenomenon. It is a common event in the metastases of neoplasms and is a normal event with chorionic tissue in pregnancy. Though most chorionic pulmonary emboli disappear the occasional rare fatal case of chorionic embolism has been reported in pregnancy. Mechanical injury of tissues can lead to embolism. We have already referred to bone marrow embolism following closed-chest massage (Figure 2.39) and crushing of other tissues such as the liver can lead to embolism of fragments of liver.

Finally, foreign body embolism is a well-documented phenomenon examples of which are fragments of wood, pins, thorns, bullets, bits of intravenous catheter and needles and fragments of cotton wool. These post-injection emboli have been described in the lungs of children and others who for one reason or another have required repeated intravenous infusions. Nowadays foreign body emboli are most frequently seen in drug

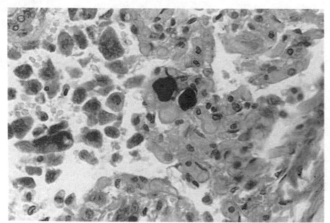

Figure 2.40 *Section of lung showing magenta-coloured corn starch particles in capillaries. This follows the intravenous injection of pulverized tablets suspended in water*

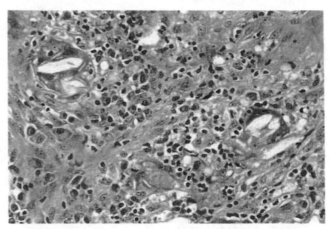

Figure 2.41 *A talc granuloma showing foreign particles of talc encompassed by foreign body giant cells*

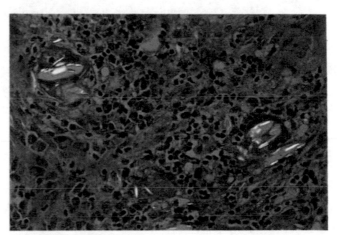

Figure 2.42 *The talc granuloma in polarized light showing the refractile talc particle*

addicts who inject themselves intravenously with a wide variety of drugs (Figure 2.40). Many of these are in tablet form so that they need to be ground up and suspended in water before injection. The water used often is taken from a lavatory pan or some other unhygienic source. It is not therefore surprising that foreign body embolism and endocarditis are frequent amongst these addicts.

The pulmonary complications of intravenous drug abuse are many and varied. An acute complication with the use of opiates such as heroin and morphine is the development of fatal pulmonary oedema. Opiate pulmonary oedema was first described by Osler in 1880 but its frequency has only been recently appreciated (this syndrome was responsible for 48% drug-related deaths between 1950 and 1961 and 80% of such deaths from 1970 to 1971 in New York City[22]. The precise mechanism is obscure but delayed or immediate hypersensitivity, neurogenic, hypoxic or direct toxic actions have been suggested.

The other possibility is that the oedema is due to adulterant substances but this is unlikely since it occurs not only with heroin but with methadone and morphine as well. The most likely factor is hypoxia due to respiratory depression leading to increased capillary permeability and consequent pulmonary oedema. It resembles in many ways the pulmonary oedema of high altitudes where pulmonary hypertension also occurs because of the pulmonary arteriolar vasospasm brought about by the hypoxia.

Later on other lesions may develop in the lung such as talc granulomatosis, sometimes called 'blue velvet' and 'red devil' lesions after the substances that have been injected. Blue velvet lesions are caused by the injection of crushed tablets of paregoric and pyribenzamine, and red devil lesions are the result of the intravenous injection of the contents of secobarbital (Seconal) capsules. In both cases the talc content of the preparations was incriminated and similar lesions have been produced by weekly intravenous injections of talc

in rabbits. Histological examination of the human and rabbit lungs reveals many talc granulomas and conspicuous endothelial proliferation of pulmonary arteries (Figures 2.41, 2.42). Repeated and prolonged intravenous injections of talc or talc-containing tablet contents can ultimately lead to a rigid lung because of diffuse pulmonary fibrosis. Rarely emphysema may result from ischaemic atrophy of lung tissue caused by embolic blockage of capillaries in many parts of the lung[23]. A number of other pulmonary complications have been reported such as thrombotic pulmonary hypertension, collapse of lung tissue, asthma, bronchopneumonia, and pyaemic abscesses.

Infective endocarditis is also a common complication of intravenous drug abuse affecting principally the tricuspid valve, causing 8.7% of addict deaths in New York City from 1950 to 1961. Some areas have a mortality as high as 70% from endocarditis following heroin abuse. The mortality depends very much on the speed and vigour with which therapy is instituted. Staphylococci and Candida are the common infection organisms though mixed infections with intestinal organisms are frequent. Septic pulmonary emboli are frequently found and often provide the basis for the initial clinical presentation[24].

The sequelae of injury are many and varied and affect a large number of people. Many are curable if diagnosed and treated early but of even more importance is the fact that a lot can be prevented.

Bibliography

1. Sevitt, S. (1970). Reflections on some problems in the pathology of trauma. *J. Trauma*, **10**, 692
2. Stehbens, W. E. (1972). *Pathology of the Cerebral Blood Vessels*, pp. 351–471. (Saint Louis: C. V. Mosby)
3. Tedeschi, C. G. (1945). Cerebral injury by blunt mechanical trauma. Review of Literature. *Medicine (Baltimore)*, **24**, 339
4. Case, M. E. S., Archer, C. R., Hsieh, V. and Codd, J. E. (1979). Traumatic aneurysm of the vertebral artery. A case report and review of the literature. *Angiology*, **30**, 138
5. Courville, C. B. (1950). *Pathology of the Central Nervous System*, 3rd Edn., pp. 296–301. (California: Pacific Press Publishing Association)
6. Johnson, R. T. and Yates, P. O. (1956). Brain stem haemorrhages in expanding supratentorial conditions. *Acta Radiol. (Stockholm)*, **46**, 250
7. Dommissee, G. F. (1974). The blood supply of the spinal cord. *J. Bone Jt. Surg.*, **56B**, 225–235
8. Campbell, R. (1981). Management of pancreatic injuries. *Hosp. Update*, **7**, 25
9. Maloney, A. F. J. and Whatmore, W. J. (1969). Clinical and pathological observations in fatal head injuries: a five year survey of 173 cases. *Br. J. Surg.*, **56**, 23
10. Strich, S. J. (1961). Shearing of nerve fibres as a cause of brain damage due to head injury. A pathological study of 20 cases. *Lancet*, **2**, 443
11. Cushing, H. and Eisenhardt, L. (1938). *Meningiomas. Their Classification, Regional Behaviour, Life History and Surgical End Results*. (Springfield Ill: Charles C. Thomas)
12. Haerem, J. W. (1974). Mural platelet microthrombi and major acute lesions of main epicardial arteries in sudden death. *Atherosclerosis*, **19**, 529
13. *The Organ in Shock*. (1977). Proceedings of the Second Symposium on Recent Research Developments and Current Clinical Practice in Shock. A Scope Publication. (Kalamazoo, Michigan: The Upjohn Co.)
14. Leader. (1977). Crush injuries. *Br. Med. J.*, **2**, 1244
15. Beyer, A. (1979). Shock lung. *Br. J. Hosp. Med.*, **21**, 248
16. Wardle, N. (1979). Bacteraemic and endotoxic shock. *Br. J. Hosp. Med.*, **21**, 223
17. Gresham, G. A., Kuczynski, A. and Rosborough, D. (1971). Fatal fat embolism following replacement arthroplasty for transcervical fractures of the femur. *Br. Med. J.*, **2**, 617
18. Jackson, C. T. and Gerendyke, R. M. (1965). Pulmonary and cerebral fat embolism after closed-chest cardiac massage. *Surg. Gynaecol. Obstet.*, **120**, 25
19. Sevitt, S. (1962). *Fat Embolism*. (London: Butterworths)
20. King, P. (1970). Fat embolism syndrome. *Med. J. Aust.*, **2**, 1190
21. Hartveit, F., Lystad, H. and Minken, A. (1968). The pathology of venous air embolism. *Br. J. Exp. Pathol.*, **49**, 81
22. Helpern, M. (1972). Fatalities from narcotic addiction in New York City. *Hum. Pathol.*, **3**, 13
23. Vevaina, J. R., Civantos, F., Viamonte, M. and Avery, W. G. (1974). Emphysema associated with talcum granulomas in a drug addict. *South. Med. J.*, **67**, 113
24. Curtis, J., Richman, B. L. and Feinstein, M. A. (1974). Infective endocarditis and drug addicts. *South. Med. J.*, **67**, 4

Chapter 3

Accidental, Suicidal or Homicidal Injury

The study of wounds is mainly directed towards relating the tissue and organ changes to the mechanisms of injury and the time of their occurrence. In itself it is a fascinating aspect of biology but this study is also the key to the assessment of the mode of death. The position, form and grouping of wounds is often of great value in determining whether they were inflicted accidentally, suicidally or as the result of homicide.

The details of various sorts of wounds and the methods involved in determining their age were described in Chapter 1. This section deals mainly with patterns of wounds and the lessons that may be learned from them.

The first step in the examination of any wound is to try to determine whether it was inflicted before or after death. This is usually not difficult because of the absence of any visible vital reaction at the edges of the wound. Retraction of the edges of wounds and other visible indications of inflammation indicate the ante-mortem origin of wounds. Post-mortem wounds have a typical parchment-like appearance with sharp clearly defined edges devoid of any inflammatory response. They can be produced in a variety of ways. Movement of a heavy body after death may lead to considerable damage to the body as it is bumped down flights of stairs or some such (Figure 3.1). The vast majority of sudden deaths are due to cardiac, cerebral or pulmonary causes and because they often occur in confined spaces the body may be injured as it collapses. One of the commonest post-mortem injuries is bruising of the nose due to a fall. This is often accompanied by extensive periorbital bruising due to flexing and stretching of the facial skin with consequent rupture of fine blood vessels (Figure 1.6). This common post-mortem injury also emphasizes

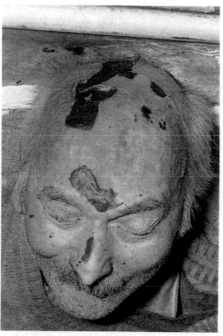

Figure 3.1 *Post-mortem abrasions caused by a fall on the face at the time of death. There is no vital reaction and the wounds have a parchment-like appearance*

that extravasation of blood can occur after death if vessels are dilated at the time of injury. Likewise the finding of blood near to a body with a scalp laceration does not imply ante-mortem injury. Here again great dilatation of vessels at the moment of death can lead to such bleeding if the vessels are injured. Agonal scalp lacerations are a frequent finding in sudden deaths from natural causes.

A number of factors influence the degree of force needed to produce a wound. This is a question that is

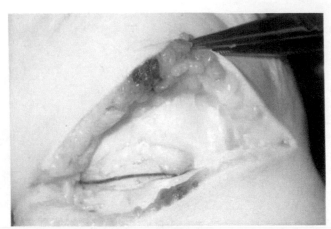

Figure 3.2 *An incised recent bruise in the subcutaneous fat of a baby. There is little surface change in skin colour to indicate the deeper bruising*

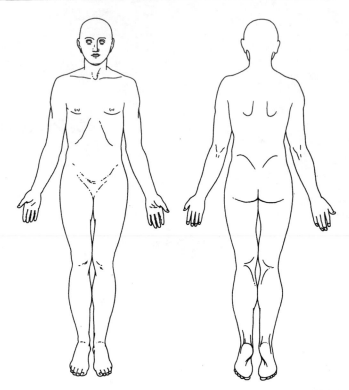

Figure 3.3 *Line drawing of a body for recording superficial injuries*

often asked of a medical witness in criminal cases and the answer must be carefully considered and suitably qualified. The very young and the aged bruise easily and a slight force can produce an extensive bruise in an old person where the skin is thin and the vessels often fragile. Bruises in babies on the other hand are sometimes difficult to see because of the abundant subcutaneous fat in these children. Such bruises may easily be missed and consequently a pattern of bruises may not be appreciated (Figure 3.2).

When giving evidence in court it is important to use terms that lay people can readily understand. It is equally important not to use phrases that may lead to prejudice. For example, when trying to explain the degree of force needed to produce a laceration in the front of the scalp it is helpful to provide alternatives. Such a wound could have been produced by a fall on the forehead, a blow with a blunt object and they are commonly seen in victims of car accidents and so on. However, when the evidence is clearly present one should not be daunted from saying that the most likely cause of a cluster of bruises on an arm was the firm grip of a hand. Clearly, proper answers to lawyers in court depend upon the accurate observations of the pathologist, his full use of all available techniques in studying the wounds, and lastly upon his experience. If any of these are deficient then he must say so.

In order to ensure an accurate record it is essential to make handwritten notes and diagrams at the scene of death both during and after autopsy. These are the sum total of the pathologist's observations and should be available for scrutiny by the court if needs be. Printed sketches of parts of the body are particularly useful for this purpose (Figure 3.3).

In the UK as in the USA only about half of those who practise the speciality of forensic pathology do so on a full-time basis. The remainder are part-time practitioners who are also engaged in routine morbid anatomy and histopathology in hospitals. For this reason it is important to recount by means of examples

some of the problems that might arise. From the start to the finish of the investigation the pathologist should always have in the forefront of his mind questions that are customarily asked by prosecutors, defence counsel and judges.

The essence of success is to proceed slowly, resisting all pressure for speed from police, in particular, who are anxious to begin their investigations once the mode of death is known. Detailed photographic records of the scene, objects around or on the body, clothing, wounds and anything else, whether it appears relevant or not, are essential[1,2].

The variety of problems that might arise can be illustrated by the death of a drug addict[3]. Death may have been due to the sudden onset of pulmonary oedema as we have already described. However, other factors such as physical assault may be associated. Or the person may have died in police custody, in a motor vehicle accident, or as a result of violent attempts at resuscitation by his own drugged colleagues who supposed him to be dead. The deceased may have been moved after death to some other place by colleagues who fear detection and their own involvement at the place of death. Sometimes colleagues burn or bury the body and burned or decomposed remains may be all that is left for examination.

The pathologist must therefore be prepared to answer questions from lay persons about identification, time of death, cause and manner of death, period of survival after injury and about types of materials such as hair, paint, powders and so on about the body.

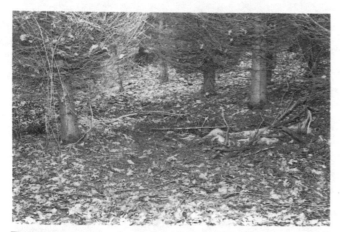

Figure 3.4 *Legs of a corpse in a coniferous wood*

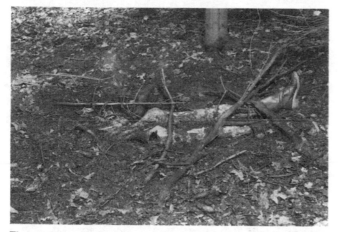

Figure 3.5 *Closer view of the legs clad in long boots with overlying branches of a deciduous tree*

It is axiomatic that the circumstances surrounding the death be known to the pathologist and he may wish to delay the performance of the autopsy for this information. Another reason for delay is that surface injuries may develop more clearly hours after death. It is also useful to look at the external appearances again after the autopsy has been done. When blood has drained from the tissues bruises may often become apparent having been invisible in congested skin before the autopsy.

Scars, tattoo marks, needle marks, operation scars all need to be recorded and special attention is paid to recording the dentition accurately. Finger printing is part of the identification procedure and can even be done on macerated or mummified skin.

Badly burned or severely decomposed bodies are the most difficult to handle and interpret. Radiographic examination of epiphyses, skull sutures and the state of ossification of costal and laryngeal cartilages will help in determining the sex and age of the body. Bodies that have decomposed in open ground are often torn to pieces by predators such as foxes. The neck structures are frequently lost in this way so that detection of changes of strangulation can be completely lost. The skull may also be separated from the body and found some distance away from the rest of the corpse. However, articles of jewellery and so forth might be found on the corpse and can assist identification.

Figures 3.4–3.8 illustrate such a case. The body of a young woman clad only in knee high boots was found in a wood in January. She had probably died there 6 months before. The head was separate from the body, one arm had vanished and a few items of jewellery were found. The skull was cleaned and revealed a good set of teeth in both jaws. There were three fractures in the skull caused by a light object such as the handle of a small hammer. The fractures were not depressed and the skull was thin suggesting light blows with a light object. The position of the fractures across the front of the face, side and back of the head suggested that they had been caused by a right-handed person. It was unlikely that the fractures had caused death. More likely death was due to strangulation but no evidence for this remained. The dental formula was recognized by the bureau for missing persons and a radiograph of the skull superimposed well on a photograph of the suspected victim (Figures 3.9–3.11).

It is also possible to determine the ABO blood group of bones using gel diffusion methods on material extracted from the spongiosa[4]. This can be compared with the suspected victim's group if known. If it is not, it can be determined by recovering erythrocytes from a stained blood film made during life as in the case of this particular girl.

Some cases of poisoning can be detected by the analysis of bone marrow of skeletal remains. The finding of amitryptyline in such a case is of interest but raises a number of problems in interpretation. There is much to be learned of drug distribution in various organs such as bone marrow and how this relates to the blood levels at death. In addition, the rate of decay of drugs in cadaveric bones needs to be determined[5].

Apart from identity, determination of the time of death is the other matter which is always of great concern to the police and to the judiciary. Much of the rest of the evidence hangs on this determination. With fresh bodies the determination of rectal temperature and degrees of livor and rigor mortis help in the assessment but all of them can only provide a rough estimate of the time of death. One of the most difficult tasks confronting the forensic pathologist is to convince police and lawyers that this is so. We shall deal with this problem in subsequent chapters that concern death in various circumstances.

Accidental and violent deaths comprise about 4% of all deaths per annum in the Western World. As a cause of death accidents contribute variously in different age groups. For example, motor-cycle accidents are a principle cause of death in the teenage male. In the elderly, accidents in and around the home provide an important cause of death.

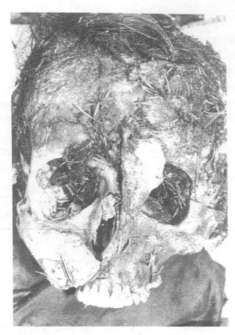

Figure 3.6 *The skull of the dead person shown in Figures 3.4 and 3.5 which was recovered some distance away from the body*

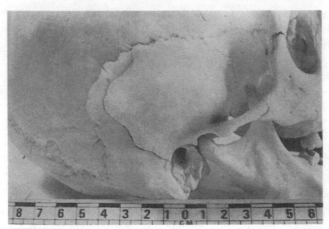

Figure 3.8 *A hair line fracture in the right squamous temporal bone of the skull shown in Figure 3.7*

Injuries caused in accidents can usually be easily recognized but injuries created by vigorous resuscitation after death may complicate the interpretation. Resuscitation attempts may result in multiple rib or sternal fractures with perforation of the lung and even rupture of the right ventricle. Injuries to the upper abdominal viscera may be caused in a similar way (Figure 3.12).

The distinction of accidental from non-accidental injury is most difficult in children that are the subjects of violence within the family. In these cases it is important to bear in mind the common accidental injuries sustained by young children. If children fall they tend to strike the various prominences of the body. Bruises found elsewhere that are said to be accidental should be regarded with suspicion. Most important are the discrepancies in the history given by those in charge of the children and the injuries that are found. Non-accidental injury to children is an important and frequent problem which we shall deal with subsequently.

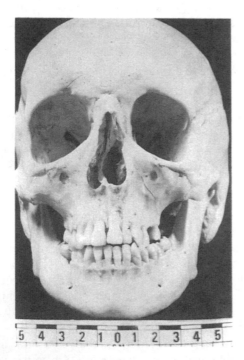

Figure 3.7 *The same skull shown in figure 3.6 after cleaning and preparation showing fractures in the left maxilla and right supraorbital ridge*

Suicide

Official statistics show that about 4000 people a year take their own lives in England and Wales and clearly this is an understatement of the incidence[6]. To get this into perspective suicidal deaths are slightly less than 20% of all unnatural fatalities and are just 0.7% of the annual morbidity from all causes. However, in the third decade of life the figure is 12.3% of all causes of death each year.

In addition to this hospitals provide care for about 2000 non-fatal suicidal attempts each week, and there are others that are not recognized as attempted suicide. Some never reach hospital at all.

In recent times the number of fatal attempts has tended to fall. This is in part explained by the change of fuel gas from coal to natural gas. However, the number of non-fatal attempts is increasing.

In order to understand the changing trends in suicidal deaths and suicidal attempts which have been regarded as distinct entities it must be realized that they have

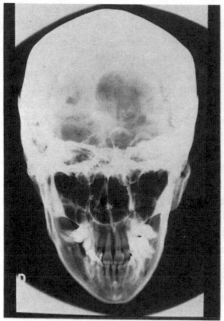

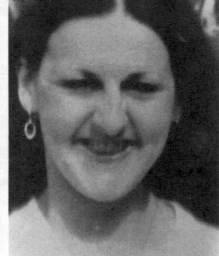

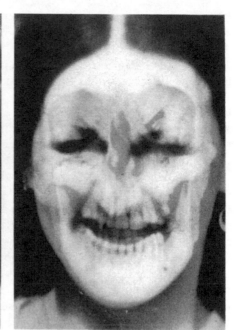

Figure 3.9 *Radiograph of the skull shown in Figure 3.7*

Figure 3.10 *Photograph of the missing person*

Figure 3.11 *Superimposition of the photograph on the skull radiograph*

been redefined as attempted suicide and deliberate self-harm. A dramatic fall in incidence occurred in England and Wales between 1963 and 1970. The crude suicide rate dropped from 121 to 80 deaths per million in that period. Furthermore, there were no compensatory increases in deaths from gassing or drowning assigned to accidental or open verdicts.

Many views have been advanced to explain this phenomenon and we shall consider some of them here. Improved knowledge of psychiatric illness and its treatment are important factors. Mental illness is a feature in 93% of cases including depressive illness (64%), alcoholism (15%) and schizophrenia (3%)[7]. A majority of these cases had consulted psychiatrists or their general practitioners within a year of death and 80% were receiving psychotropic drugs. In this context the reduction in deaths in the 1960s showed some relationship to the widespread and often successful treatment of patients with these drugs.

Other forms of treatment of suicidal attempts in ambulances and hospital emergency departments seemed to have contributed to this decline. A strong case has also been made[8] for the help given by Samaritans in promoting the decline of the 1960s. Some have contended this view because the steady decline in the suicide rate ceased at the start of the 1970s in spite of the continued growth of the Samaritan services until 1975.

We have already alluded to changes in the availability of deadly poisons as a possible factor in the decline of suicidal deaths. Highly toxic coal gas first became available in England and Wales in the nineteenth century for lighting public places. It was introduced into the home at the start of the twentieth century first for lighting then for heating and cooking. Between 1912

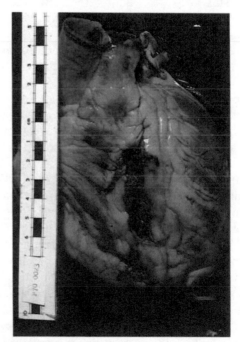

Figure 3.12 *Rupture of the right ventricle due to resuscitation attempts. The lack of bruising or any vital reaction indicates a post-mortem injury*

and 1958 the death rate from suicidal poisoning by domestic gas increased from 5 to 67 per million for males and from 2 to 51 per million in women.

In 1948 when the gas industry was nationalized the gas was produced from coal, and contained 10–20% of carbon monoxide. In the 1950s gas was produced from oil and the concentration of carbon monoxide fell to about 1%.

By 1971 nearly 70% of gas supplied came from natural gas which has practically no carbon monoxide in it.

Kreitman[9] has related the fall in fatal suicides to the steady reduction of the carbon monoxide content of domestic gas.

There are several critics of this hypothesis but the interesting observation was that with the decline of this deadly gas in the 1960s there was no change to other lethal agents. It is difficult to escape the conclusion that the rapidly lethal effect of carbon monoxide was responsible for the conversion of deliberate self-harm to suicidal death.

It is difficult to disentangle from the multitude of cuts, bruises, lacerations, fractures and poisonings those that are deliberate non-fatal self-harm and those that are accidental. This is particularly difficult in the young. Since 1961 there as been a substantial increase in the number of poisonings recorded each year. 86% of these are in persons 15 years or over. Of course it includes accidental overdose, abnormal drug reactions, cases of drug addiction such as methadone poisoning and possibly a few attempted homicides. However, a number of cases of deliberate self-poisoning are not recorded so that it now appears that there are now at least 20 cases of deliberate non-fatal self-harm for every fatal suicide. This ratio was about 6 to 1 after the Second World War. This rate of increase appears to have occurred mainly in young people.

The reduction in prescriptions for barbiturates between 1964 and 1974 accounted for a decline in suicides due to these dangerous drugs. However, the increased incidence of non-fatal self-poisoning has been accompanied by the use of other drugs such as analgesics, other hypnotics and psychotherapeutic agents and alcohol is increasingly found as an associated poison.

Methods of attempting suicide vary in different age and ethnic groups and also vary with social class and sex. They also tend to change over the years. For example, suicides by firearms and particularly with shotguns were a feature of East Anglia in the 1950s. This method has become rare and has been displaced by self-poisoning which is a reflection of the availability of many drugs such as tranquillizers, hypnotics and analgesics, notably paracetamol and distalgesic which contains paracetamol and dextropropoxyphene.

If autopsies are done on all sudden and unexpected deaths a small proportion of unsuspected suicides are uncovered. A Danish study of 807 medicolegal deaths where the police have not asked for autopsy revealed differences in the mode of death in 4%[10]. Cases of concealed suicide were found particularly in the older age group. This is not surprising because such cases, even after autopsy, can be attributed to sudden death from coronary artery disease. No such discrepancy was found in cases of homicide. However, even in such cases it may be difficult when exotic poisons (q.v.) of one sort or another are used.

The acquisition of a detailed history and account of the scene of death is a vital essential in the discovery of unsuspected suicide deaths. A visit to the scene by the pathologist may also be necessary to be sure that agents of potential self-injury have not been overlooked or concealed by the deceased or relatives. The histories of those dying from asphyxial inhalation of stomach contents following alcohol consumption are littered with accounts of bottles of drink concealed beneath mattresses and so on. A high index of suspicion is necessary in pathologists in undertaking autopsies on any case of sudden unexpected death.

When death is due to unsuspected self-poisoning there may be little to find at autopsy. The smell of alcohol, cyanide or other aromatic poison may be detectable when the corpse is opened but may easily be missed particularly by the inexperienced. There may be tablet material visible in the stomach, often there is not. It is important always to be suspicious when pulmonary oedema of moderate degree is the only finding. It is all too easy to attribute this to left ventricular failure from ischaemic heart disease. If, however, there is no evidence of cardiac dilatation, in particular of the left ventricle, then other causes of oedema of the lungs must be considered. A common cause is some intracranial disease of one sort or another. In cases of suicide due to poisoning by hypnotic drugs the oedema is due to paralysis of either the vasomotor or respiratory centres in the hind brain. Respiratory paralysis with accompanying hypoxia is a potent cause of increased permeability in all blood vessels leading to oedema.

It might be considered wise to advise a toxicological analysis in all cases of sudden death where the cause is not easily apparent. This is an expensive procedure and more important can lead to distressing delay for relatives in the disposal of the body. When analysis appears to be inevitable then the pathologist should make sure that he retains all the necessary specimens. He may, even so, wish to advise the coroner that disposal should be by burial and not cremation. It must be emphasized that cases of this sort are rare and can be avoided by a detailed autopsy and the preservation of appropriate samples.

The specimens needed for toxicological analysis vary from case to case and from one analytical laboratory to another. It is hardly surprising to say that all samples should be taken with chemically clean ladles and syringes into clean containers. Blood from a peripheral vein should always be collected into a plain bottle and one containing sodium fluoride in a concentration of 10 mg per ml of blood.

It is unwise to take heart blood or pooled blood from the pleural sacs as this may be contaminated with stomach contents. The object of adding sodium fluoride to a blood sample is to prevent enzymatic breakdown of any alcohol that may be present. It is also important to store all specimens at +4°C to prevent decomposition products from contaminating the specimen. For example, a blood sample stored at 20–25°C for 2 days may generate up to 100 mg/dl of alcohol due to fermentation by fungi, bacteria and enzymes.

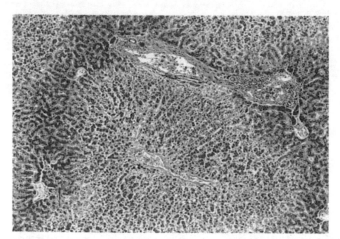

Figure 3.13 *Section of liver from a person who died of paracetamol poisoning showing extensive centrilobular fatty droplets*

In addition to blood, specimens of urine, liver and brain should be preserved. It is always wise to preserve the contents of the stomach and intestines as well. In some cases of suspected opiate poisonings in such persons as drug addicts bile is useful. Morphine is excreted in the bile and is more readily detected there than in the blood.

All samples should be carefully labelled to ensure identity and handed to the responsible officer who should provide a signed receipt for them before taking them to the laboratory. Histological examination can also reveal toxic effects of drugs on the kidney, liver and other organs. In every case representative samples of major organs should always be taken into 10% formal-saline for this purpose. For example, the delayed toxic effects of a drug like paracetamol can be detected by microscopy of the liver (Figure 3.13).

The majority of cases of suicide are easy to detect from the scene and at the autopsy. The presence of a 'suicide note' at the scene may be helpful as well. This is not infallible and cases of unsuspected homicide may be concealed.

The autopsy findings on suicidal deaths produce a variety of modes. A study of 162 suicide autopsies from 1957 to 1977 carried out in north-west London is typical of the general experience in the United Kingdom[11]. 20% revealed significant physical disease but the majority belonged to a relatively younger physical group.

Three principal methods of suicide were identified, namely drug poisoning, carbon monoxide poisoning and physical injury. During this period 890 deaths were caused by drug poisoning of which 60% was due to barbiturates and 68% were females. Most of the remainder were due to other agents, predominantly analgesics and antidepressant drugs. A few were due to cyanide and corrosives such as acids and alkalis. 603 were due to carbon monoxide poisoning and physical self-destruction was present in 369. 77% of these were males and the methods used varied. They included shooting, stabbing, slashing, drowning, hanging, falling and burning. The instruments used in such methods of physical

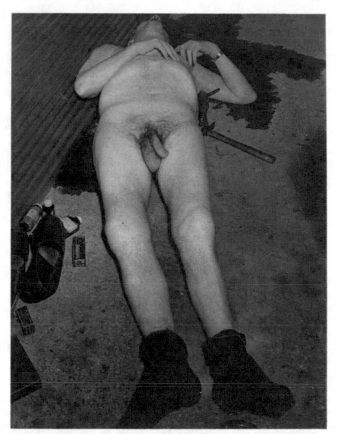

Figure 3.14 *A home-made gun lying beside the body of a man who shot himself through the base of the brain*

self-destruction are many and varied.

Suicidal shooting can be accomplished with conventional weapons such as rifles, pistols and shot-guns. Occasionally the weapon is home-made. A man found naked and dead in his garage had shot himself via the mouth through the hind brain. The weapon consisted of a piece of metal tubing held in a pair of locking pliers. A 0.22 bullet had been inserted into the tubing and discharged by tapping it with a hammer (Figure 3.14).

Suicide using conventional firearms usually occurs at point-blank range and the entry hole provides the features that confirm this. There is blackening, burning, abrasion and laceration of the skin and, in the case of double-barrelled shot-guns the abraded mark of the undischarged barrel can often be seen (Figure 1.14). Even when the discharge is at point-blank range it is important at the scene and at the autopsy to determine that the individual could have shot himself (Figures 3.15, 3.16). The position of the weapon in relation to the body and agonal abrasions on the finger that pulled the trigger are useful guides to suicidal killing (Figure 3.17).

Occasionally unusual weapons are used; perhaps the use of a cross-bow is one of the most exotic. A young man was found dead with the shaft of the bolt (arrow) of a cross-bow projecting from his upper abdomen. It had penetrated the sternum and the heart. The wound produced is of characteristic triradiate shape conforming

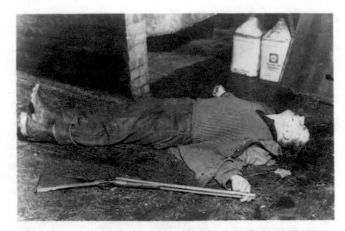

Figure 3.15 *Scene of suicidal shooting. The gun is held in the left hand and the wound is to the left side of the head. The appearances suggest a self-inflicted wound*

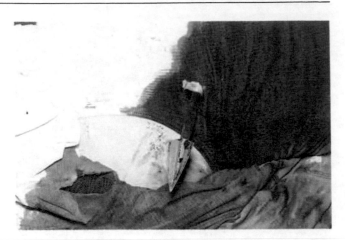

Figure 3.18 *Bolt of a cross-bow projecting from the lateral abdominal wall*

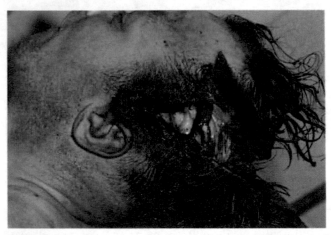

Figure 3.16 *Shot-gun wound to the left side of the head of the man shown in Figure 3.15*

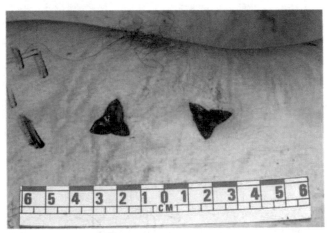

Figure 3.19 *Triradiate wounds reflect accurately the shape of the head of the bolt*

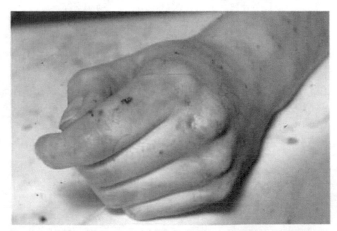

Figure 3.17 *Agonal abrasions on the forefinger caused by recoil of a shot-gun used in suicide*

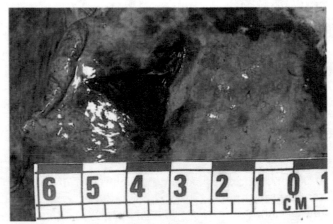

Figure 3.20 *A similar wound in the lung showing the shape of the head of the cross-bow bolt*

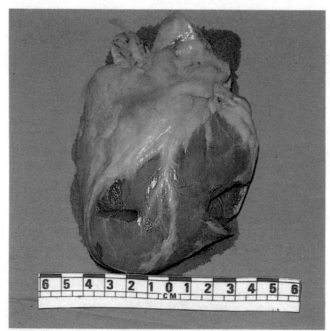

Figure 3.21 *Entry and exit holes of the bolt in the heart. The exit hole is much larger with a missile of relatively low velocity*

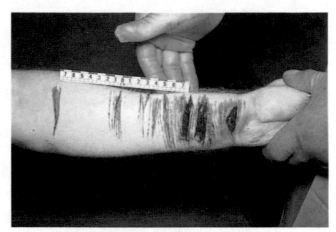

Figure 3.23 *Multiple cuts of the forearm in attempted suicide; they tend to avoid the large lateral arteries*

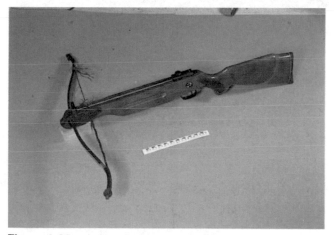

Figure 3.22 *A 'Wildcat' cross-bow*

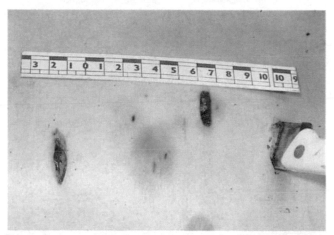

Figure 3.24 *Multiple stab wounds with a bread knife. Some are tentative stabs and show bruising indicative of a vital reaction*

to the shape of the arrow head. It had finally impaled a vertebral body and the lengths of the three cuts produced by the triradiate end provide a clear assessment of the angle of firing[12]. In order to achieve such bony penetration the speed of the bolt must have been of the order of 220 km per hour. This deadly silent weapon is fortunately rarely used to kill people. One other case of homicide with a cross-bow has been recorded[13] (Figures 3.18–3.22).

Suicide by stabbing and slashing is no longer a common event in Britain. There has been a good deal written in the psychiatric literature on the person who attempts suicide by cutting the wrists. Wrist cutters tend to be young single women and men and whilst the injury is rarely fatal it can generate a good deal of reaction from people in the environment. Razor blades, glass and knives tend to be used. The injury is usually to the left wrist indicating the preponderance of right handedness. The cuts are multiple starting with tentative knicks and finishing with deeper wounds that may severe nerves and tendons but large limb vessels at the wrist usually escape injury[14] (Figure 3.23). The small superficial tentative wounds grouped alongside the deeper ones are a strong indication of self-inflicted injury. Wrist cutting in older age groups tends to be part of a spectrum of injuries which end in death. Examples are an elderly man who cut both wrists, attempted to hang himself and eventually stabbed himself to death with a bread knife (Figure 3.24). Another middle-aged wrist slasher killed himself by jumping from a fifth floor window.

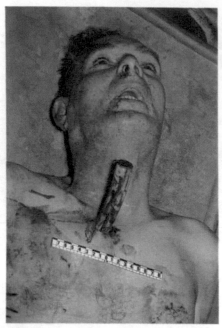

Figure 3.25 *Suicide with a kitchen knife driven down through the suprasternal notch into the aorta*

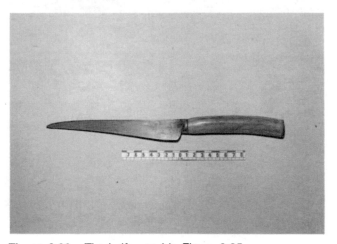

Figure 3.26 *The knife used in Figure 3.25*

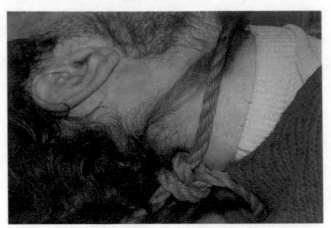

Figure 3.27 *Suicidal hanging with a nylon rope. The suspension point is at the back of the head*

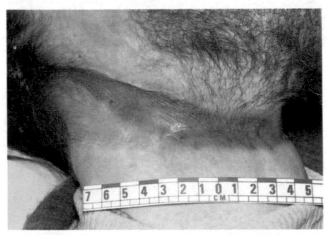

Figure 3.28 *Ligature mark from the person shown in Figure 3.27. Note the parchment-like quality of the mark*

Suicide by stabbing is not a common event. A typical mode is by driving a knife almost vertically through the skin over the suprasternal notch into the heart (Figures 3.25, 3.26). Stabbing is seen more often in homicidal deaths and has become more frequent in recent years.

Hanging remains a frequent mode of suicide. A variety of ligatures such as ropes, belts, straps, cloth and the like are used. A stout nylon rope is often employed (Figures 3.27, 3.28). The body is often not suspended above the ground and the feet frequently touch it. Sometimes the body is suspended at an angle to the ground. These deaths always raise the problem of intent: the question being whether the motive was self-destruction or sexual gratification. The application and tightening of a ligature can lead to rapid death from cardiac dysrhythmia before the individual has time to

free himself. The person depicted in Figure 3.29 died in this way having used an unusual elastic ligature which he could not loosen.

When death has occurred rapidly the post-mortem findings may be scanty. The usual indications of asphyxial death such as petechiae on the eyelids, behind the ears and elsewhere are often absent. Fluidity of the heart blood is only a measure of sudden violent death and does not necessarily indicate asphyxia specifically[15]. If the body is suspended the ligature mark usually indicates a suspension point behind an ear or at the nape of the neck (Figures 3.30–3.32). However, in the case illustrated in Figure 3.29 no such point was found, the appearances of the ligature much resembling that seen in homicidal rather than suicidal strangulation.

The ligature mark rapidly assumes a glossy brown semi-translucent appearance after death. It is rather parchment-like in its consistency. Microscopically there is squashing and fraying of the epidermis and superficial dermis representing a combination of abrasion and compression due to the ligature (Figures 3.28, 3.33).

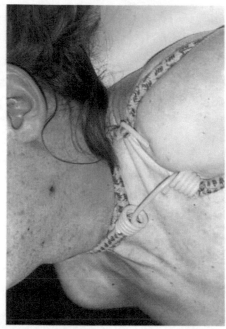

Figure 3.29 *Self-strangulation with a carrier strap. Note petechial haemorrhages in the skin above the ligature indicating that death was not immediate*

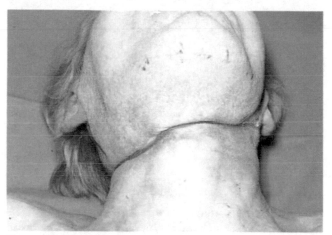

Figure 3.30 *Ligature mark rising to a suspension point below the left ear*

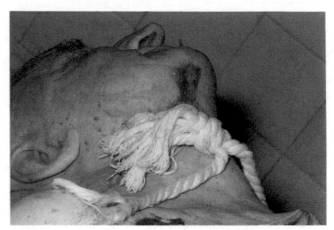

Figure 3.31 *Ligature with a suspension point below the chin*

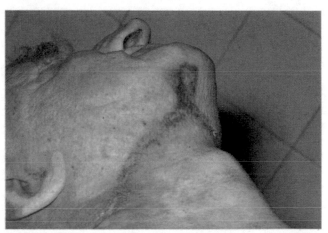

Figure 3.32 *Same case as Figure 3.31 with the ligature removed*

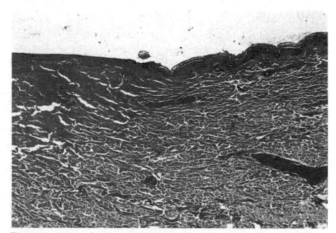

Figure 3.33 *Section of ligature mark showing epidermal compression*

It is wise to be aware of the possibility of other causes of death in persons who appear to have died from self-strangulation. Not infrequently high concentrations of alcohol or other drugs may be found in the blood and the question then arises whether the final act of strangulation by the ligature was self-induced or not. Usually the findings at the scene help to resolve this problem.

Asphyxial death can also result from placing plastic bags over the head. Polythene sheets and bags are hazardous because they are tough and waterproof. They are excellent containers but placed over the head they can be lethal. Accidental suffocation is particularly common in children playing with these things and putting them over their own heads or that of a playmate.

It can also occur in those indulging in auto-erotic practices. Most of such cases are recorded in the German literature. Plastic bags have also been used to assist intoxication by addicts using anaesthetic or narcotic vapours such as glue solvents. Homicidal suffocation by the use of plastic bags is very rare but it is also difficult to detect because the classical signs of asphyxial death may be absent. The only suspicion is aroused by finding a little pulmonary oedema and some regurgitation of stomach contents into the air passages[16].

Suicidal suffocation with a plastic bag can be achieved by the bag alone or in combination with the inhalation of carbon monoxide or other toxic gas and vapour. Polson and Gee[16] report four cases. They encountered the first in 1961. Two were by suffocation alone. Of the other two one had a high blood alcohol and the other was under the influence of the barbiturate (sodium amytal) and alcohol.

Some deaths usually occur in obvious circumstances. Many show signs of asphyxia and no other evidence of injury. The presence of drugs, evidence of sexual deviant behaviour and the presence of disease that may have prediposed to suicide must be carefully sought for.

Moisture inside the bag is often due to water exuded from the body after death and does not necessarily imply that breathing had occurred whilst the head was inside the bag. Even a cushion in a plastic bag will exude water when warmed. It is for this reason that paper bags rather than plastic bags are desirable for the transportation of exhibits such as clothing to the forensic science laboratory.

When asphyxial changes are not found the mechanism of death may be doubtful. Sometimes the bag is sucked into the mouth and causes immediate cardiac and respiratory arrest. In other cases the bag is sucked over the nose and mouth forming a rapid and effective seal of the air passages.

Suicide by drowning presents similar problems to those encountered with self-strangulation. Sudden immersion in cold water may be rapidly fatal and again the problem of intent arises. In these cases other factors such as high blood alcohol or other drug levels might contribute to death. Sometimes certain articles of clothing such as shoes, handbag, umbrella and so on are left on the river bank before entering the water. This and the occasional finding of a note of intention will help to confirm the diagnosis of suicide. Suicidal drowning in waterways is not uncommon in rural areas. Drowning in a bath is rarely if ever suicidal and some other cause for death under such circumstances must be sought for. Other causes are likely to be drugs, carbon monoxide poisoning derived from incomplete combusion of gas in a geyser in the bathroom or by electrocution. We shall say more of this when considering deaths in the home.

In cases of drowning there is often little to find at autopsy. The lungs may be moist but the most reliable indicator that the person was alive on entering the water is the presence of water gulped into the stomach.

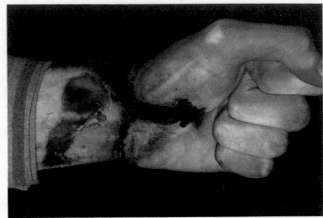

Figure 3.34 *Suicidal electrocution. Wires around the wrists were connected to a mains plug. Note charring of the palm and desquamation of the skin of the wrist*

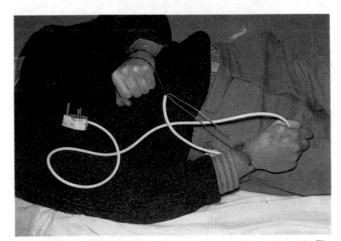

Figure 3.35 *Method of suicidal electrocution shown in Figure 3.34*

Prolonged immersion is followed by decomposition and marks of violence may disappear because of this. For example, ligature marks of strangulation may be difficult to find. Microscopy of the skin taken from suspicious areas will help to clarify this issue. Likewise analysis of blood may be of no value in such a body. However, the vitreous humour is the least likely to be affected by decomposition and this should be collected for the determination of alcohol and other drug levels.

A few other indications of drowning might be found such as a rise in magnesium levels in the vitreous humour after drowning in sea water. There may be microscopic evidence of disseminated intravascular coagulation after drowning in fresh water. Asphyxial haemorrhage into the middle ears and mastoid air spaces provides strong evidence of drowning[17].

Electrocution is usually an accidental event. Occasionally it forms a method of suicide (Figures 3.34, 3.35). Usually the entry and exit marks of the current are easy to see and this is particularly easy when it is suicide because the individual when found is often still connected to the current supply. Histological examination of tissues at suspected sites of electrical injury may

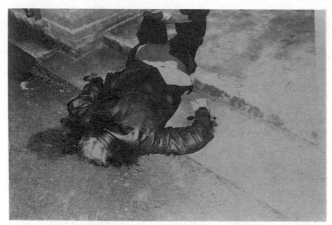

Figure 3.36 *Severe head injuries in a man who jumped from a five-storey window*

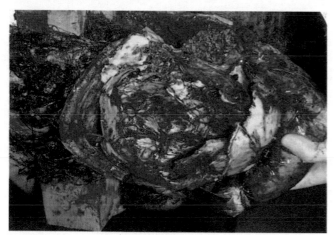

Figure 3.37 *Comminuted skull and lacerated brain from the man shown in Figure 3.36*

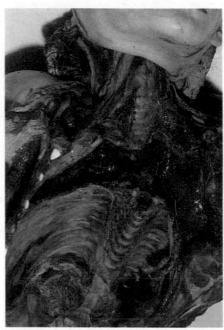

Figure 3.38 *Fracture dislocation of the thoracic spine following collision with a train*

reveal some evidence. There may be tiny intraepidermal blisters, vasothrombosis and tearing of elastic fibres in the walls of small blood vessels.

Self-burning is a rare event. It occasionally occurs in times of political strife when a person ignites his petrol-soaked body as a gesture of defiance against oppression. People are sometimes consumed by fire in car accidents and it has been suggested that some single-car, single-occupant road deaths are suicidal. A study of 528 such cases in Great Britain (1969 and 1970) revealed a seasonal variation. The road deaths were maximal in November whereas suicides had a peak in April. The road deaths were more frequent in the young whereas suicides increased with age. The conclusion was that whilst some of the road deaths were intentional, the numbers involved were too small significantly to affect the suicide rate in general[18].

Collision with the ground or with moving vehicles is occasionally intentional. Jumping off tall buildings is a mode employed by those determined to kill themselves. These are probably a different psychiatric group from many who make suicidal gestures. Damage to the body is severe (Figures 3.36, 3.37) involving multiple fractures and organ ruptures associated with severe decelera

tion injury. If a body falls from a height and lands on its back the body splays open. Severe distraction fractures occur in the pelvis and thorax and organs such as the heart, lung, spleen and kidneys may be wrenched from their attachments and lie free in the body cavities.

Collision with vehicles can result in severe injury, as for example a body that has been struck by a train. It is not unusual for mentally ill persons to wander on to rail tracks and lie in front of an oncoming train. The consequences are obvious. The head may be cut off or the body transected (Figure 3.38).

The variety of devices that can be used to produce deliberate self-harm are infinite. This relates to the ingenuity of man to create ways of self-destruction or to adopt established devices such as new solvents, motor vehicles and the like for that purpose. A remarkable case of self-injury by a middle-aged man who drove nail-sets into his head is such an example. His wife heard him hammering in his workship and subsequently found him with about one inch lengths of the nail-sets protruding from his scalp. He subsequently recovered after surgery despite the dangerous proximity of the instruments to the superior sagittal sinus[19].

Homicide

Man is an unusual creature, being distinguished from the rest of the animal kingdom by his propensity to kill, maim and torture his own species. When considering the matter it is important to use the term homicide rather than murder or manslaughter because these are specific legal terms. Thus it is that the incidence of homicide is increasing whereas murder is declining. This merely reflects current legal practice.

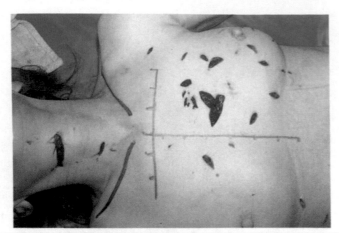

Figure 3.39 *Multiple stab wounds of varying shape produced by direct stabbing and twisting of the knife on withdrawal. A slash cut across the neck is often seen in such cases*

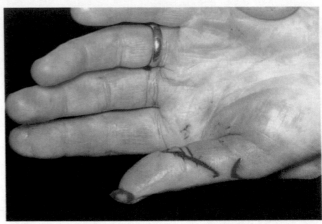

Figure 3.40 *Cuts in the thumb. These are defence wounds caused by the victim trying to grab or to ward off the knife*

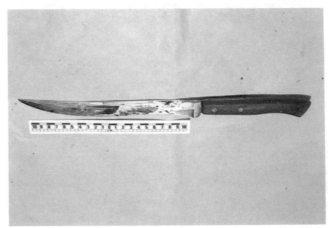

Figure 3.41 *A kitchen knife used for stabbing. It is important to record the dimensions of the blade and handle and any stains upon them*

Homicide has been with us ever since records of human activity were preserved. It has always been a popular subject and has formed the basis of plays, operas and novels for many years. Mass murderers have always attracted attention and many of these are legendary, the stories being a popular mixture of violence, suspense and horror. Mass murderers are defined as those who kill more than one person over a period of time. This situation in particular results in the mobilization of the entire force of forensic experts in order to achieve a solution.

In mass murders the mode of killing tends to be repetitive. Every aspect needs careful record and study. The circumstances, such as the time of day, place, method of injury and the degree of force needed to effect it are all important. Often the same type of victim is selected. Jack the Ripper in the last century and the more recently convicted Yorkshire Ripper both selected female victims, who were women of similar age who they believed to be prostitutes[20,21].

Homicide, whether mass killing or otherwise, may be spontaneous or planned. Most are spontaneous, and are the result of family dispute, lovers' arguments and the like. The ingestion of alcohol is often a provocating feature of the situation. When the mentally ill kill people solution of the cause can be difficult for the motive is often obscure[22]. Religious rivalry and nationalistic fervour result in killings that cannot easily be attributed to one killer. Problems of this sort exist in Northern Ireland at the present time. We shall deal with these injuries in a chapter on civil strife.

The precise legal definition of homicide becomes more difficult in cases of probable euthanasia. The killing of severely abnormal infants either by positive action involving the administration of drugs or negative withdrawal of life-supporting measures is a recurring problem. Many of these deaths occur in hospital and a variety of techniques are employed[23]. Examples are air embolism, injections of insulin, curare, potassium chloride, succinyl choline and so on. Life support is withdrawn by switching off ventilators, withholding antibiotics, tampering with the oxygen supply to ventilators and other means.

In some of these cases the argument centres on the definition of irrecoverable disease and ultimately on the criteria for the establishment of brain death. This matter is being actively debated in the United Kingdom at the present time. People argue that the criteria of brain death apply only to the vital centres in the hind brain but are no indication of the presence or absence of cortical activity. This is a serious and almost insoluble problem which reflects greatly on those involved in the transplantation of hearts and livers, which are only of value if removed from a body at the moment of defined death.

Patterns of wounding are of great importance in the investigation of homicide and they tend to be similar from case to case. Stabbing, for example, is often multiple, usually to the breast area and often features slash wounds across the front of the neck (Figure 3.39). This pattern coupled with defence wounds on the hands is the hallmark of homicidal stabbing (Figure 3.40). The weapon used is often the one that come most easily to hand: a whole range of kitchen knives have been found at various scenes of murder (Figure 3.41).

In a series of 28 persons charged with murder the weapon used was improvised in 16 cases. The remainder comprised shooting, strangulation and poisoning[24]. In this sense also the majority of those aged 40 or over were judged to be criminally insane and most of these had a family history of psychiatric illness. Murder in the setting of a stable marriage was a sure indication of severe mental illness. The rest of these cases included schizophrenia, depressive illness, a mixed paranoid group and several with severe personality disorder. The paper concludes with a strong plea for the Prosecutor to seek a verdict of insanity rather than to oppose it because this resulted in longer detention of the person with greater protection of society. Parker[25] pursues a similar theme in his series of 100 persons accused of murder or attempted murder. He found a considerable proportion were mentally ill or severely emotionally disturbed and that at least one in ten murders could have been prevented. He stresses the need for more careful assessment and treatment of potentially violent psychiatric patients.

The incidence of homicide is increasing and the methods of accomplishing it change. A study from Cuya Loga County which includes the city of Cleveland has revealed some important facts about this[26]. Previous studies in Cleveland had shown that homicide was related with poverty, an intimate acquaintance between victim and assailant and a preponderance of non-white victims. These aspects were reviewed in the recent study from 1938 to 1971, a period encompassing the middle third of the 20th century[26].

The results are interesting because the criteria for the verdicts of homicide and suicide in this jurisdiction were consistent since one man had been the Coroner since 1936. In the latter part of the 1960s the homicide rate rose more rapidly both in the County and in the City of Cleveland. Suicide rates also increased during this period though the trend was slight compared to the rise in homicide. In the first part of the period under survey firearms were involved in 50–60% of homicides. In the latter part of the time guns accounted for 80% of the victims. 90% of these were produced by handguns and this indicates the need for a radical review of the law governing the possession of firearms in the USA.

Following homicidal assaults bodies are often concealed, mutilated and dismembered and all the skills of forensic science are needed to unravel the case. The Ruxton case of 1935 is a classical example. Dr Ruxton had killed his wife and a nursemaid. The bodies had been neatly dismembered by disarticulation, teeth had been extracted and the terminal phalanges of the hands cut off. This method of dismemberment pointed to an individual with a knowledge of human anatomy and forensic practice. Despite the fact that at least 70 pieces of human remains had been scattered over a wide area they were reassembled and identified. Particular note

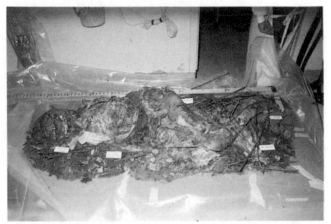

Figure 3.42 *Decomposed remains of a murdered woman found 6 months after her disappearance*

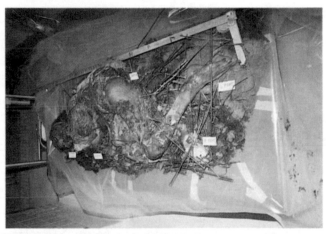

Figure 3.43 *Some parts of the body are recognizable and labels are attached to identify them and their position in relation to the earth on which the body lay and which had been removed with the body*

was made of the superimposition of photographs of the deceased persons on radiographs of the skull[27]. Ruxton was convicted and hanged.

Reconstruction of the skeleton is an important part of the process of identification and can be extremely difficult if mutilation is severe (Figures 3.42, 3.43). In general, when assembling the pieces it is easier to aim for reconstruction of a lateral rather than a frontal view[28]. Radiographs of all skeletal remains may reveal old injuries or evidence of disease and a careful examination of all pieces of skin is essential (Figure 3.44). This may reveal material for finger printing, birthmarks, old scars and tattoo marks. Amongst the skeletal fragments the pelvis is particularly useful in determining the sex of the person if no other evidence remains (Figures 3.45, 3.46). The most reliable index which correlates with the sex in 90% of cases is the greater sciatic notch/acetabular index. The index is computed by dividing the width of the notch by the vertical diameter of the acetabulum and multiplying by 100. In general, pelves with an index of more than 88 will be female. Those with an index of 86 or less are likely to

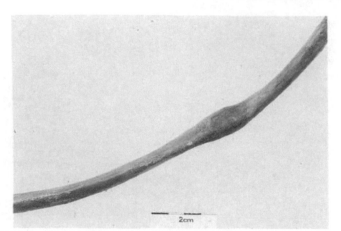

Figure 3.44 *A ninth rib from the subject shown in Figures 3.42 and 3.43 showing a healed fracture. This assisted identification by comparison with radiographs taken in life*

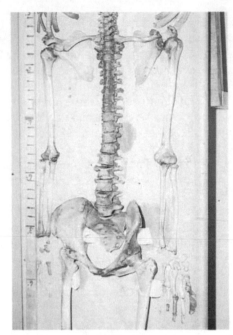

Figure 3.45 *The assembled skeleton enabling limb bone measurements to be made to determine height*

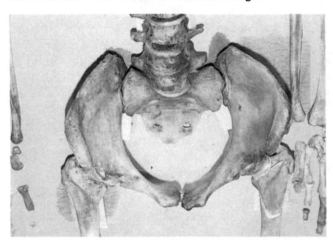

Figure 3.46 *The pelvis showing typical female configuration*

be male. This index is particularly useful when the pelvis is fragmented[29].

Blood stains may still be present on the remains and it is possible to learn a good deal from dried blood. There are well-developed methods for grouping these stains. Thus it is possible to detect antigens of the ABO, Rh and MN groups. In addition, allotypic markers, Gm_1, Gm_2 and Inv_1, can be detected on γ-globulin molecules together with several blood groups of the polymorphic enzyme and protein systems of red blood cells and serum.

Other methods may subsequently prove to be of value in forensic work. Sex can be determined by the detection of differential fluorescence of the leukocyte Y chromosome in the presence of magnesium chloride. The age of the blood stain can be guessed at by changes in the spectrophotometric features of the blood pigments and maternal blood stains can be identified by the detection and quantitation of chorionic gonadotrophin[30].

Sometimes the teeth are the only remains that enable victims of homicide to be identified. This is particularly true after incineration of the body. There are few practitioners of the art of forensic odontology but the field is growing rapidly as new techniques are added to methods of dental identification.

The obvious application is in the matching of the dental formula of the dead person with one of the centrally held records of missing persons (Figure 3.47). Dental histology can also help in placing the approximate age of the individual. Criteria that are used for this estimation comprise attrition, gingival recession, secondary dentine, cementum root resorbtion and root transparency[31]. Identification plates bearing details of the individual can be planted into teeth when they are filled. We shall say more of this when considering identification of persons involved in aircraft disasters.

Human bite marks have been important evidence in cases of homicide and rape in recent years. They also feature occasionally amongst the wounds inflicted during non-accidental injury to children. If the bite

includes a substantial proportion of the dental arches the task is relatively easy. The identification of an assailant from dental marks on a piece of chewing gum found at the scene of death is a more unusual aspect of forensic odontology. Food can also provide traces of blood or saliva both of which may help in identification. 80% of the population secrete blood group substances in saliva and other fluids such as sweat, tears and semen[32].

We have already said that violent crime against persons is increasing. In the USA from 1960 to 1968 the rate (per 100 000 persons) of reported robberies increased by 119%, aggravated assault by 67%, rapes by 65% and homicide by 36%. In 1968 sexual assaults were 5% of these crimes of violence and the incidents included rape and molestation of children[33]. The possibility of rape must always be considered in cases of female homicide and the appropriate tests need to be done.

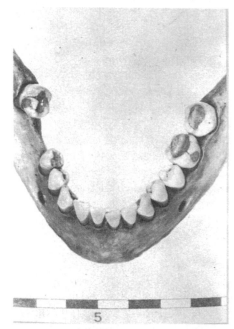

Figure 3.47 *The lower jaw of the body shown in Figure 3.42. Comparison of the dental work with a record of dentition of missing persons enabled precise identity to be established*

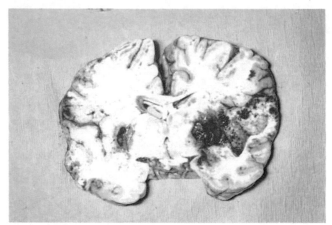

Figure 3.48 *Multiple brain haemorrhages making it difficult to decide whether trauma was the sole cause or whether one of the haemorrhages was due to natural causes*

Those who survive rape may be taken to any practising physician but it is wise to refer the task to doctors, such as police surgeons, who are practised in dealing with such problems[34]. The interview and examination should proceed along the lines of any other consultation. Consent of the victim and the presence of a chaperone are mandatory. The prime objective is to determine whether the alleged incident occurred. In other words, did recent intercourse occur and was there evidence of violence? It may not be possible to answer either of these questions. A second aim is to establish prior or existing conditions which may have been aggravated by the assault. For example, the presence or absence of mental illness and a negative pregnancy test which may later become positive and therefore be associated with the rape.

A good history should record the time, place and circumstances. The examination should record general appearances of the clothes and the body and any evidence of a struggle. Abrasions, lacerations, stab wounds and bruises should be recorded and radiology done where bony injury is suspected. The external examination of the genitalia must be made methodically. A vaginal speculum can be used except in children and young virgins to look for evidence of laceration, pregnancy, discharge and bleeding.

Laboratory samples should include fluid aspirated from the posterior fornix. It can be examined for sperm by a wet preparation and by a Gram stain which will also show organisms such as *Neisseria gonorrhoeae*. Microbial cultures should be done. The fluid can be examined for the presence of semen by a test for acid phosphatase. Finally blood for serology will help to

exclude syphilis and urine for gonadotrophins will exclude pregnancy. A subsequent examination 4 weeks later may detect emotional upset, venereal disease or pregnancy.

The collection of fully representative material from such cases of rape is essential. The doctor should not rely on the prompting of police but must act on his own initiative. A survey of medically obtained evidence at incidents of sexual assault revealed woeful inadequacies[35]. Failure to obtain clothing of the victim precluded the finding of useful evidence such as fibres, hair, dust, grease, plant materials and dried blood. Dried blood stains on the body must also be collected together with samples of pubic hair, head hair and finger-nail scrapings. As well as vaginal swabs it is useful to have anal and oral swabs if the subject allows. Victims may be reluctant to admit to oral sex though they may have been forced to do it as part of the act of rape.

It is wise, therefore, in rape as with the examination of other cases of violent crime to have a protocol which must be followed rigidly. The use of a prepared kit for sample collections is especially helpful in the management of suspected sexual assault.

One of the most difficult problems facing the forensic pathologist is to assess the part played by a fight, a struggle or an assault in the death of a person. This occurs when, for example, the wounds received are relatively slight and clearly of themselves are not fatal. Even so the individual may drop dead at once or die some days later. Figure 3.48 illustrates a coronal slice of brain from a 60-year-old man who was attacked and fell to the ground. He sustained a parieto-occipital fracture and contusion to the parietal cortex and temporal poles of the brain. These injuries were revealed by a CAT scan when he was admitted to hospital unconscious. However, the scan also revealed a haemorrhage into the external capsule of the brain. This is a site for spontaneous haemorrhage and had occurred at the time of the affray. Before the event he had no evidence of neurological abnormality. Afterwards he developed

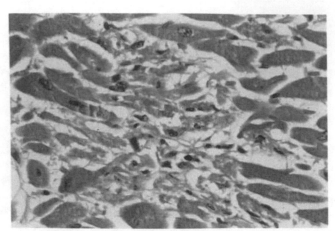

Figure 3.49 *Foci of dying cardiac muscle cells with an inflammatory response. Such lesions are seen after some intracranial damage*

signs attributable to the spontaneous haemorrhage. He subsequently died and autopsy revealed extensive surface necrosis of the brain and the presence of a small spontaneous external capsular haemorrhage. Such small haemorrhages are an occasional incidental finding at necropsy and have not always led to death.

Several questions arise in a case of this sort. First, was the spontaneous haemorrhage precipitated by the fight? Second, would it alone have been fatal or was the surface injury contributory? Third, how were the skull fracture and the surface brain injury caused? Was it the result of a fall due to the spontaneous haemorrhage or did it result directly from the fight?

The problem is virtually insoluble. The man's heart weighed 260 g and histological examination of organs did not reveal any evidence of pre-existing hypertensive vascular disease. It is likely therefore, but difficult to prove, that the spontaneous haemorrhage could have been the result of a sharp rise of blood pressure during the assault. On the evidence available it was decided not to press charges.

Stress cardiomyopathy is another vexed problem with wide implications. It is difficult to prove the hypothesis that the cumulative effects of psychological stress and pain can kill. However, one rare group of homicidal deaths provides a reasonably credible model in support of the hypothesis of lethal stress. There are individuals who are virtually beaten to death and yet the injuries alone do not provide a satisfactory explanation of the lethal outcome. A study of 15 homicide victims who were beaten to death showed that 11 had foci of myofibrillar necrosis in the subendocardial parts of the left ventricle with variable degrees of inflammatory cellular infiltration (Figure 3.49). In those that survived a few days after the assault cardiac dysrhythmias such as atrial fibrillation, a variety of tachycardias and a wandering pacemaker were found[36]. Similar changes have been reported in persons dying of intracranial haemorrhage[37] and lesions have been produced experimentally using long-acting sympathomimetic agents such as isoprotorenal[38].

The myocytolysis is most likely due to focal coronary arterial spasm produced by catecholamines released during stress. Hypothalmic stimulation produces similar effects in experimental animals.

Not only does this 'stress cardiomyopathy' explain death in persons with otherwise non-lethal injury but it also raises other problems as well. As we have already said a variety of intracranial catastrophes may result in myocytolysis. Some of these people are maintained on respirators and may be candidates for cardiac donation as transplants. This adds another factor to the debate surrounding the ethics of such transplant operations and emphasizes the need for careful scrutiny of the quality of the hearts that are used.

Bibliography

1. Gresham, G. A. and Turner, A. F. (1979). *Post Mortem Procedures*. (London: Wolfe Medical Publications)
2. Ludwig, J. (1979). *Current Methods of Autopsy Practice*. (Philadelphia, London, Toronto: W. B. Saunders Co.)
3. Gross, E. M. (1972). Preparation for court. *Hum. Pathol.*, **3**, 97
4. Kellermann, G. (1971). Methodological investigations on the ABO typing of ancient bones. *Humangenetik*, **14**, 50
5. Noguchi, T. T., Nakamura, G. R. and Griesemer, E. C. (1978). Drug analysis of skeletonising remains. *J. Forensic Sci.*, **23**, 490
6. *Suicide and Deliberate Self-Harm*. Office of Health Economics, Number 69, January 1981
7. Barraclough, B. M., Bunch, J., Nelson, B. and Sainsbury, P. (1974). A hundred cases of suicide: clinical aspects. *Br. J. Psychiat.*, **125**, 355
8. Bagley, C. R. (1968). Samaritans and suicide. *Soc. Sci. Med.*, **2**, 1
9. Kreitman, N. (1976). The coal gas story. United Kingdom suicide rate, 1960–71. *Br. J. Prev. Soc. Med.*, **30**, 86
10. Asnaes, S. and Paaske, F. (1980). Uncertainty of determining mode of death in medico-legal material without autopsy – a systematic autopsy study. *Forensic Sci. Int.*, **15**, 3
11. Gatter, K. and Bowen, D. A. Le. (1980). A study of suicide autopsies 1957–1977. *Med. Sci. Law*, **20**, 37
12. Sivaloganathan, S. and Devlin, J. W. A. (1979). Suicide by a quarrel. *Police J.*, **52**, 42
13. Gresham, G. A. (1977). Arrows of outrageous fortune. *Med. Sci. Law*, **17**, 239
14. Harris, C. N. and Rai, K. (1976). The self-inflicted wrist slash. *J. Trauma*, **16**, 743
15. Gresham, G. A. (1978). Violent forms of asphyxial death. In Mason, J. K. (ed.), *The Pathology of Violent Injury* (London: Edward Arnold)
16. Polson, C. J. and Gee, D. J. (1972). Plastic bag suffocation. *Z. Rechtsmed.*, **70**, 184
17. Sammut, J. J. (1967). The middle ear in accidental deaths. *J. Laryngol. Otol.*, **81**, 137
18. Jenkins, J. and Sainsbury, P. (1980). Single car road deaths – disguised suicides? *Br. Med. J.*, **281**, 1041
19. Fox, J. L. and Branch, J. W. (1971). Intracranial nail sets. An unusual self-inflicted foreign body. Case report. *Acta Neurochir.*, **24**, 315
20. Historical Forensic Cases. The Jack the Ripper Murders. (1981). *Inform*, **13**, 2

21. American Mass Murders. The Forensic Aspects. (1981). *Inform*, **13**, 2
22. Leader. (1973). Dangerous Patients. *Br. Med. J.*, **1**, 247
23. Hospital Crimes and Hazards. The Forensic Aspects. (1981). *Inform*, **13**, 2
24. Medlicott, R. W. (1976). Psychiatric aspects of murder and attempted murder. *NZ Med. J.*, **555**, 5
25. Parker, N. (1979). Murderers: a personal series. *Med. J. Aust.*, **1**, 36
26. Hirsch, C. S., Rushforth, N. B., Ford, A. B. and Adelson, L. (1973). Homicide and suicide in a Metropolitan County. *J. Am. Med. Assoc.*, **223**, 900
27. The Ruxton Case. (1973). In Rentoul, E. and Hamilton Smith (eds.), *Glaister's Medical Jurisprudence and Toxicology*, p. 90 (Edinburgh and London: Churchill Livingstone)
28. Drake, W. and Lukash, L. (1978). Reconstruction of mutilated victims for identification. *J. Forensic Sci.*, **23**, 218
29. Kelley, M. A. (1979). Sex determination with fragmented skeletal remains. *J. Forensic Sci.*, **24**, 154
30. Divall, G. B. (1974). The characterisation of blood stains in forensic science. *Lab-Lore*, **6**, 321
31. Maples, W. R. (1978). An improved technique using dental histology for estimation of adult age. *J. Forensic Sci.*, **23**, 764
32. Sperber, N. D. (1978). Chewing gum – an unusual clue in a recent homicide investigation. *J. Forensic Sci.*, **23**, 792
33. Hayman, G. R. and Lanza, C. (1971). Sexual assaults on women and girls. *Am. J. Obstet. Gynaecol.*, **109**, 480
34. Burges, S. H. (1978). The role of the police surgeon in sexual offences. *The Practitioner*, **221**, 737
35. Weaver, R. L., Lappas, N. T. and Rowe, W. F. (1978). Utilisation of medically obtained evidence in cases of sexual assault: results of a survey. *J. Forensic Sci.*, **23**, 809
36. Cebelin, M. and Hirsch, C. S. (1980). Human stress cardiomyopathy. Myocardial lesions in victims of homicidal assault without internal injuries. *Hum. Pathol.*, **11**, 123
37. Feibel, J. H., Campbell, R. G. and Joynt, R. J. (1976). Myocardial damage and cardiac arrhythmias in cerebral infarction and subarachnoid haemorrhage: correlation with increased systemic catecholamine output. *Trans. Am. Neurol. Assoc.*, **101**, 242–244
38. Hill, R., Howard, A. N. and Gresham, G. A. (1960). The electrocardiographic appearances of myocardial infarction in the rat. *Br. J. Exp. Pathol.*, **41**, 633–637

Chapter 4

Injury at Work

The severity and nature of industrial injuries vary with the type of job involved. In the steel industry where people are handling heavy, hot objects there is much danger and injury and strict codes of practice need to be provided and complied with if the hazards are to be avoided. The maintenance of a register of all injuries is essential but equally important is a register of incidents which do not involve personal injury but are still a potential hazard. Registers of this sort tend to reflect constant patterns of injury. For example, minor cuts are a steady feature of accident reports in histological laboratories. Accident and incident registers are the basis for improved patterns of work that should reduce injury at work.

A more subtle form of work injury is caused by exposure for varying periods of time to chemical substances of various kinds. Claims for compensation for such industrial diseases must show that the individual was exposed at work. They must also show that the substance concerned produces deleterious effects which have reduced the life span or capabilities of the individual. The adverse effects are many and variable ranging from a shortened life span, reduction of physical ability to more subtle but still incapacitating psychological disturbances.

The determination of a cause and effect relationship of an industrial agent is not always simple. The particular agent responsible may not always be present and may disappear from the industrial environment altogether as practices in the processes used change. The effects of the agents may also be modified by factors such as the mode of exposure, the presence of other synergistic agents and the susceptibility of the individual.

A wide variety of chemical substances may be found in various industrial processes. Many of these substances may enter the body and are metabolized or excreted by the breath, skin, urine or faeces. Some of them like the silicate and carbon dusts are retained in the lung and lymph nodes, other substances are stored in bone, body fat and keratin of skin, hair and nails. The dose needed to produce toxic effects may be large such as coal dust which may be as much as 100 g in a miner's lungs. On the other hand, small amounts such as 0.5 g of chrysotile asbestos may produce pulmonary asbestosis.

A long period may elapse before hazardous substances produce their effects. This is particularly true of carcinogenic compounds which may take 10–20 years to produce neoplasms.

Agriculture

Farming is one of the more dangerous occupations as was emphasized by Cooper[1] in 1971. In 1967 the Ministry of Agriculture, Fisheries and Food reported 8686 accidents and diseases in agricultural workers in England and Wales. Of these 1.3% (114) were fatal. The major causes are machines, animals, falls, wounds and poisoning.

Accidents on the farm tend to involve the elderly and the young. A farm abounds with hazards for the unwary or the partially sighted and unsteady. Farming is hazardous because the worker is often required to handle a wide variety of pieces of equipment, some of which are cumbersome and very heavy. It is not surprising that overturned tractors in ditches and the like provide one of the commonest and most serious of farm accidents (Figure 4.1). Long irregular hours and unfavourable, often badly lit, conditions of work are strong predisposing factors to accidents on the farm. Dusty conditions, contamination with manure and so on add to the complications of wounds that occasion such accidents. Gas gangrene and tetanus are obvious examples of particular infectious hazards in the farm environments[2].

69

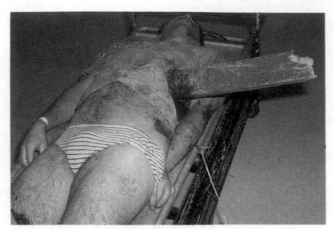

Figure 4.1 *A lorry overturned and impaled the driver on a fence. Overturning vehicles such as lorries and tractors are especially hazardous on the farm*

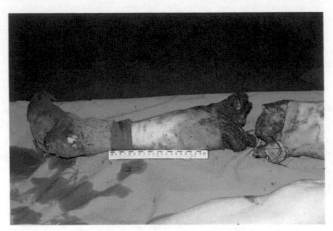

Figure 4.2 *Avulsion of the lower leg caught in a drive shaft on a farm*

Many farm implements can produce injury. The tractor is the most common and if a driver is injured when the machine overturns he has a one in four chance of being killed. The lethal properties of these machines are partly due to their high centre of gravity making them unstable on rough ground and partly due to the strength or lack of it of the protective cab and the driver of the vehicle.

Sweden was the first European country to devise safety cab regulations in 1959 and required that all new tractors for agricultural use should have strong safety frames. Basically the safety frame is required to fulfil several criteria for adequate safety. The cab must be strong and there should be no dangerous internal projections that might injure the driver. Visibility from within should be good and the level of noise should not be so high that the driver is unaware of things going on around him outside the machine. Measures of this sort have significantly reduced the number of deaths in Swedish agricultural practice.

The tractor is also used as a stationary source of power for moving other agricultural machines. This is done by means of the so-called 'power take-off' which is a rapidly rotating shaft. Entanglement of clothing in such an unguarded shaft can lead to severe avulsion injuries of limbs (Figure 4.2).

A host of implements such as circular saws, vehicles with tailboards and tow bars are found in agriculture and in many other industries. The patterns of injury that may occur are obvious and need not be dwelt on here. Attention should, however, be directed to an implement that causes severe mangling injury if suitable precautions are not taken. In agriculture it is used as a grain auger which propels grain along a shaft by the turn of a screw. A similar machine is used for processing certain types of shell-fish in the fishing industry. As with most pieces of equipment safety is assured if the specified precautions are taken. Inadequate instruction or reckless behaviour can be fatal.

Animals on the farm provide a special hazard emphasized by Steele-Bodger[3]. Lacerations, crush injuries,

falls and sprains can all result from animal handling. Bulls are the most unpredictable of farm animals and the commonest species to injure the farm worker. Pigs, horses and bullocks also take their toll. Contrary to popular belief, injuries caused by cattle are not usually due to goring with horns but are usually due to the weight of the animal. The victim is often trampled upon or crushed by the kneeling animal. The extensive crush injuries can resemble those due to vehicular injuries. If the person is found dead and the animal has left the scene the only clues as to the cause of the accident may be the footprints and hairs of the creature on the corpse. Apart from such injuries, falls from horses remain one of the commonest serious sport injuries in this country.

Farm injuries are particularly prone to be complicated by tetanus infections. This is well known; nevertheless in Cambridge only 9% of 57 patients attending with open wounds inflicted in agriculture had been fully immunized against the disease. There are other infections associated with agriculture but they are surprisingly rare. Fungal infections of the skin due to Trichophyton species are occasionally acquired from cattle. Cattle ringworm in man can be a severe, unpleasant condition affecting the scalp or other keratinized areas (Figure 4.3). Leptospiral infections from contact with water contaminated with rat urine might be expected to be frequent. No more than about a dozen deaths from this disease occur in England each year. The risk of contracting Weil's disease occurs in other industries where rats and water come into contact with people. It is a recognized risk in shallow coal mines and is recognized as an industrial hazard warranting compensation. Notable outbreaks of infection in the past have been in fish markets where water and rats are abundant.

Toxic chemicals litter the agricultural scene, weed killers and pesticides being the most prominent of these. Many of these substances are also used in domestic gardens and we shall deal with chemicals such as paraquat under the heading of injuries in the home (Chapter 6).

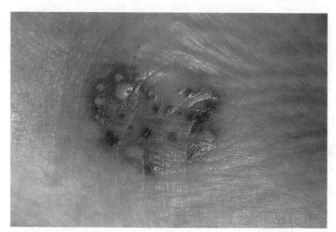

Figure 4.3 *'Ringworm' caused by Trichophyton verrucosum, a fungus acquired from contact with infected cattle*

Pesticides are often sprayed from aircraft and accidents have occurred with these by mechanical collision with pylons and the like. The pilot of the plane is peculiarly vulnerable to pesticides if proper precautions are not taken during the process of spraying. Accidental overexposure to organophosphorus pesticides can lead to changes of emotional tone and affect probably due to changes of limbic activity and disturbance of the cholinergic parts of the reticular formation. Such exposure caused a pilot to crash his aircraft on landing. He survived and subsequent clinical and biochemical studies revealed that the likely cause of the accident was pesticide poisoning[4].

The more general effects of pesticide contamination have been widely discussed in recent years. This is especially so in the case of the organochlorine compounds which can enter the body by food, air and water and are widely disseminated in the environment by biological food chains. The presence of pesticide residues in places remote from their original sites of application indicates the likely extent of the problem. Residues have been detected in wildlife in the Antarctic and in sea birds in the Pacific. Migrating fish, birds and wind and water can distribute these substances over the surface of the earth. They can also have effects on marine phytoplankton reducing their powers of photosynthesis.

Organochlorine compounds are highly soluble in lipids. Since 1964 the amount of these substances in human body fat has declined due, no doubt, to a reduction in the usage of these substances. This is encouraging and many now hold the view that the potential dangers of these compounds are no less than the indiscriminate use of antibiotics or the presence of naturally occurring fungal toxins in the environment[5].

Injury at sea

Workers at sea and off the shores of the United Kingdom comprise a large and important part of the labour force of the UK. Many work in the fishing industry and in recent years workers in the oil industry have increased considerably. Fatal accidents amongst fishermen vary in incidence from year to year depending upon the number of ships lost at sea. However, the rate can be at least twice that in the coal mining industry and 20 times that for those working in manufacturing processes.

Fishing from trawlers is one of the most hazardous occupations. Conditions are crowded, the hours are long, rough weather makes work difficult and the abundance of nets, winches and other gear all predispose to frequent injury and loss of life.

The range of injury is wide and comprises falls in heavy weather and trauma to limbs and legs from entanglement in winches, ropes and other gear. Even handling fish themselves can cause dermatitis and wounds from scales, teeth and spines. Skin conditions are very common amongst trawler workers, about one man in five being affected. Constant movement of the ship makes the engine room, galley and trailing electrical equipment more dangerous than in other circumstances[6].

The continued development of offshore gas and oil exploration has created a new field of medicine. Whilst doctors have long been familiar with the problems of divers working at depths, the complexities of these new offshore operations raise many more problems associated with diving. The introduction of deep-sea oxyhelium diving has created the need for new knowledge about the effects of increased densities of helium on thermal balance, notably respiratory heat loss and the various manifestations of acute decompression sickness[7].

The process of obtaining offshore oil and gas involves the erection of oil rigs and the laying of pipes to convey the products to the land. Men working on the drilling deck sustained most accidents which occurred during the handling of heavy equipment. Falls, crush injury and blows from moving objects produced injuries most often. Clearly the role of the crane driver of the rig is important as any misjudgement on his part can produce serious injury to a number of the crew.

Injuries to the hands are particularly common in members of the drilling crew connecting pieces of pipe and in those handling pipes on the barges that lay them.

Diving techniques have been in use for some time as a form of 'sub-aqua' sport. Their uses in industry need to be modified in relation to the type of work and the depths at which it has to be done. The main risk to any diver is a sudden change of pressure. The pressure of water increases by 101 kPa for every 10 m of depth. With increasing depths the volume of air needed to fill the lungs increases. Any sudden ascent to normal atmospheric pressures can result therefore in overdistension of the lungs. In addition, nitrogen which has dissolved in the blood because of the increased partial pressure may form bubbles on rapid decompression. This and tearing of the distended lung may lead to gas embolism affecting the brain and the spinal cord with severe results such as quadriplegia.

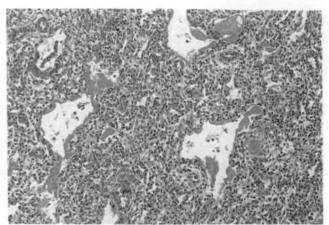

Figure 4.4 *Section of lung showing pink hyaline membranes lining alveoli following administration of high concentrations of oxygen*

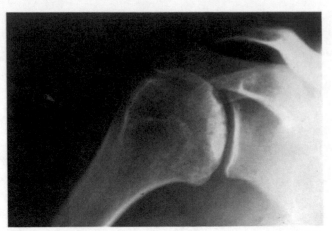

Figure 4.5 *Dense areas of necrotic bone in the head of the humerus*

Four main diving techniques are in current use by divers in the offshore oil industry. The details of these methods are recounted elsewhere: suffice to say that they are all designed to allow work to occur in circumstances that present adverse effects[8].

The pathological features of pressure change have already been partly indicated. In detail they comprise dysbarism which is the expansion or compression of gases in confined spaces such as the chest, accessory nasal sinuses and the middle ears. The term decompression sickness describes the effects due to release of bubbles of gas into the tissues from solution in the body fluids. The term 'bends' has often been used loosely to describe these two conditions. Its most satisfactory use is to describe the effects of decompression sickness on the musculoskeletal system giving pain in the limbs and the rest of the skeleton.

Increased pressure also alters the toxicity of oxygen and nitrogen. Oxygen inspired at pressures greater than 303 kPa gives rise to fits. There are no pathological features detectable in the nervous system. Breathing hyperoxic mixtures at lower pressures damages the Type 2 pneumocytes of the lung. Surfactant production is impaired and hyaline membranes form in the alveoli (Figure 4.4). Continued exposure to the hyperoxic mixture leads to septal fibroblastic proliferation and hyperplasia of alveolar lining cells. Oxygen toxicity is probably involved in other causes of this adult syndrome of respiratory distress such as persons treated on artificial ventilators.

Nitrogen under pressure also produces adverse effects, notably a sense of confusion and loss of judgement. Replacement of nitrogen by helium in the inspired air prevents this nitrogen narcosis. Being less dense than air, helium alters the speed of sound and the pitch of the diver's voice rises considerably. This can make communication difficult.

Fat embolism has occasionally been recorded in fatal decompression. There is a well-recognized association between intravascular bubbles of gas, globules of fat and the presence of disseminated intravascular coagulation. The source of the fat is controversial and cannot be explained solely by disruption of adipose tissue by gas bubbles.

An association between human fat embolism and intravascular coagulation has been reported by many investigations. There has been much debate whether the coagulation was due to trauma rather than being specifically associated with fat embolism. Soloway and Robinson[9] used intravenous triolein in rabbits and claimed no association with fat embolism and a coagulation disorder. However, the association in decompression disease may indicate that some causal association exists. It is not reasonable to propose that the presence of gas or fat in the microcirculation might provide turbulent or arrested flow leading to platelet aggregation. This is no mere academic argument. If air or fat embolism are associated with intravascular coagulation the use of heparin might be valuable therapy. The autopsy procedure on persons dying of suspected barotrauma is a special affair. It is essential not to introduce air during the procedure nor to allow post-mortem decomposition to take place by delaying the autopsy. Post-mortem radiography is valuable in showing a pneumothorax or evidence of dysbaric osteonecrosis which may develop months or years after pressure exposure (Figure 4.5). The common sites are the neck of the femur and humerus and upper end of the tibia. Subcutaneous emphysema of the neck and chest may be palpable where pulmonary barotrauma has resulted in rupture of the lung and facial lividity and petechiae may be found. Vessels leading to and coming from each major organ should be tied before cutting. The organs can then be opened under water before the feeding vessels are opened. The presence of air in the unopened vena cava is strong evidence of venous gas embolism[10].

Mining

After oil exploration and deep sea fishing mining is the most important high-risk occupation in causing injury

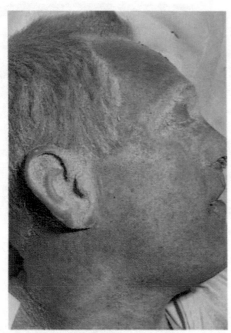

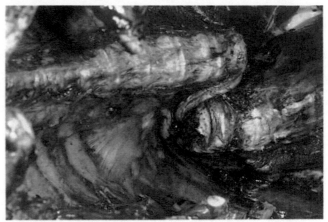

Figure 4.7 *Crush injury of the thoracolumbar region with fracture dislocation of the spine and avulsion of the spinal cord*

Figure 4.6 *Congested face with abundant petechial haemorrhages from a man trapped by a fall of grain in a store*

and death in the UK. Hazards of mining have been greatly reduced in the past 50 years and though major disasters are less because of improved pit construction, relatively minor injuries have fallen but little to the present day. Death and injury are much more frequent in coal miners than in those working in other mines. This probably reflects the preponderance of coal mining in the UK and the fact that the operation occurs at greater depths than other forms of mining and quarrying.

Coal cutting machines have precluded the need for miners to work directly at the coal face so that severe spinal injuries from falls of rock are less common than they used to be. Occasional injuries of this sort occur and severe traumatic asphyxia can occur when the body is trapped by a fall of finely divided coal or rock. This sort of injury involves trapping of the chest which stops breathing and occurs in other industrial processes (Figure 4.6). Severe congestion and large crops of petechial haemorrhages and ecchymoses are seen along the pressure line. It is implicit that the individual must have survived for a few seconds at least for the haemorrhages to develop.

The use of various sorts of machinery in the pit leads to a variety of injuries which are no different from those sustained by those who work with vehicles on rails or other vehicles. Nicoll[11] pointed out the traumatic lesions that tend to be peculiar to coal miners. There are injuries due to falls of rock or coal leading to hyperflexion of the spine. This causes crush injuries of the vertebral bodies particularly in the thoracolumbar region. The crush injury may be so severe as to rupture the posterior interosseous ligament. Damage to the spinal cord or cauda equina produces paraplegia all too frequently (Figure 4.7).

Fires and explosions in coal mines are fortunately not frequent. They occur from sparks generated by electrical or other equipment leading to the ignition of methane or finely divided coal dust that falls out from between the major coal seams. Mixtures of air and methane, which is present in all sorts of coal both hard and soft, are highly explosive when about 10% methane is present. Coal dust in the atmosphere can also lead to explosions and a mixture of methane and dust is particularly dangerous. Ignition of the gas leads to combustion of the dust and this flame spreads at great speed along the tunnels in the mine followed by a blast wave which travels more slowly. Under these circumstances death is due to burning or asphyxia by carbon monoxide formed in the confined spaces or both.

Minor hazards of coal mining have been greatly reduced by mechanization of the coal retrieving process underground and by the provision of such things as baths at the pit head. In the 1930s men left the mine in the same state as they came to the surface. Bathing and washing was done at home in cramped conditions with an insufficient supply of hot water. It is not surprising that infections of the hands, knees and elbows traumatized by the work are common. These conditions of 'beat' hand, knee and elbow are frequent; sometimes the swellings are due to bursitis as well.

Inhalation of coal dust itself is not always disabling. Other factors complicate the issue such as the presence of silicon dioxide in the coal. Hard coal is more likely to cause trouble than the soft variety. In Wales the problems are greater in the anthracite mines of the South than in the lignite, soft coal mines in the North of the province.

Respiratory disability was often called 'the dust' in North Wales. This was not always due to inhalation of coal dust. Associated chronic bronchitis and emphysema related to smoking were often important contributory factors. The incidence of tuberculosis and other respiratory infections was also frequent in the 1930s. Some individuals do show a peculiar sensitivity to coal

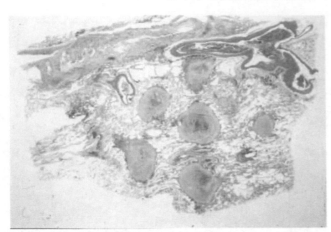

Figure 4.8 *Low power view of a section of lung showing scattered nodules of fibrosis due to inhalation of silicon dioxide*

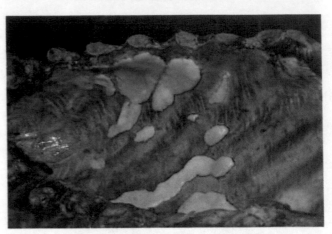

Figure 4.9 *Raised, white, fibrous plaques from asbestos exposure. This man worked in the electrical industry. Such plaques are visible radiologically*

dust giving rise to progressive massive fibrosis of the lung. This is to be distinguished from silicosis where interstitial deposits of silicon dioxide lead to nodular fibrosis of the lung and associated infection (Figure 4.8). The peculiar tendency of silicon and also asbestos dusts to predispose the lung to tuberculosis infections is well known. Early work on this matter was done by Kettle and others in Cardiff. The association of silicaceous disease of the lung with various industries is perpetrated in the names – miner's rot, potter's rot, flint knapper's rot and so on.

Whilst many of the older well-known industrial diseases are being eliminated by protective measures and legislation new ones arise. There are about 15 000 chemical and physical agents being used in industry at the present time and many new ones enter the industrial scene each year. Unfortunately the hazards of these substances are not readily recognized because of the long latent interval that may occur between exposure and effects appearing. The use of experimental animals to detect deleterious side-effects is not always reliable because of considerable variations that may exist in species response to the agents.

Harmful substances can enter the body by inhalation, ingestion or through the skin. We have already referred to industrial exposure to silicon dioxide but it is not only those directly involved in the industry who may be affected. Workers in other parts of the plant, nearby residents and even workers' families may be affected by dusts in the environment.

A large number of organs can be affected by industrial poisons. However, the bulk of lesions tend to occur at the principal portals of entry, namely the air passages, gut and skin.

Asbestos and its related diseases provide a good example of the many problems associated with exposure to industrial poisons. The term asbestos covers a range of minerals containing silicate existing as fibres which are capable of splitting into smaller fibrils. There are several forms of which crocidolite (blue asbestos) seems

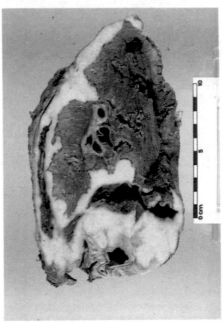

Figure 4.10 *Greatly thickened pleura by a mesothelioma extending into the interlobar fissure*

to be the most dangerous[12]. Diffuse mesothelioma of the pleura is a neoplastic accompaniment of asbestos exposure. No case of mesothelioma in Britain has implicated any other form of asbestos than the blue variety.

Asbestos is a physically strong substance and is resistant to the effects of heat and corrosive substances. Its insulating and absorbtive capacities have led to a wide application of the substance in industry. It has some 3000 uses such as tiling, piping, insulators, sealing material, fire blankets and curtains, filters and so on. The dust enters the lungs and the aortic lymphatics and may cause fibrous reactions in the interstitium of the lung and in the pleura (Figure 4.9). Its association with mesothelioma has been mentioned which may occur 30 years or more after exposure. The degree of exposure may be slight. It appears as white fleshy masses encasing the lung (Figure 4.10). Histologically it can assume an

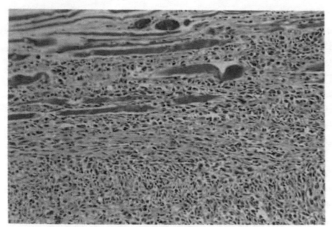

Figure 4.11 *A mesothelioma invading diaphragmatic skeletal muscle. The cells are nearly all of the spindle variety*

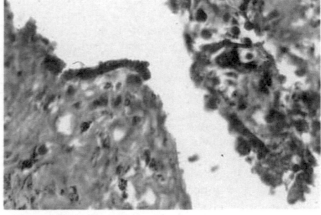

Figure 4.13 *Asbestos bodies in a section of lung. They are brown in colour*

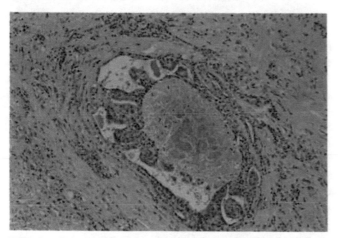

Figure 4.12 *Mesothelioma composed of papillae clothed with cuboidal cells. The neoplasm is invading a blood vessel*

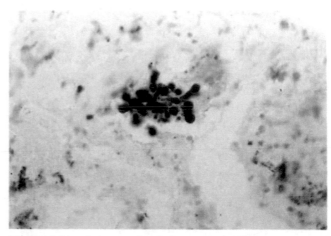

Figure 4.14 *Asbestos bodies stained by the Prussian blue method for ferric iron. They stain blue*

epithelial or sarcomatoid form (Figures 4.11, 4.12). The tumour usually invades locally but it may spread to distant organs. It may also affect the peritoneal cavity encasing the abdominal organs. The association of bronchial carcinoma with asbestos exposure is even more important and this is greatly enhanced by cigarette smoking.

The essential property of asbestos is its ability to form fibres; a fibre being defined as a particle which is at least three times as long as its width. These fibres may subdivide to form particles of molecular size on to which a variety of substances may be absorbed such as Mg, Ca, Fe, carcinogenic agents and so on. Fibres which are more than $5\,\mu$m wide cannot enter the lungs. Smaller ones divide up into components which are as little as 15 nm in diameter. The important feature of these small objects is their large surface in relation to the small mass.

The precise mode of events leading to fibrogenesis by the asbestos fibre is not yet elucidated. The first reaction in the lungs is a response of alveolar macrophages which together with erythrocytes collect around the fibre and become enmeshed in reticulin fibres. Small

particles of asbestos are phagocytosed by macrophages, larger ones are surrounded by macrophages which form a foreign body giant cell. The cells ultimately degenerate to form an asbestos body with the fibre at its central core coated with haemosiderin derived from erythrocytes and also with proteoglycans. These asbestos bodies, also called ferruginous bodies, stain blue with the Perl's method for haemosiderin and this is a useful way of showing them in histological preparations (Figures 4.13, 4.14). They vary in size from 10–60 μm long and 0.5–25 μm in width. They are only rarely found outside the lung. They are occasionally seen in the tracheobronchial lymph nodes and sometimes even further afield in thyroid, kidney, spleen and liver[13].

Not all ferruginous bodies contain asbestos and these must be distinguished from true asbestos bodies if the proper incidence is to be assessed. Asbestos inhaled into the lungs tends to drift towards the pleura via the lymphatics and pass downwards towards the lower lobes. This explains the occurrence of plaques on the inferior pleura and fibrosis and malignancy in the lower lobes of the lungs.

A number of views have been proposed to explain

the pathogenicity of asbestos fibres. The fibre itself has been incriminated because of the metals deposited on its surface or merely because of its specific size and shape. Associated factors have also been implicated in producing fibrosis such as infections and auto-allergy. Antinuclear antibodies have been found to be elevated in cases of asbestosis.

The degree of exposure to asbestos required to produce pathological changes may be slight. This is disturbing because individuals may be involved who have no direct contact with the mineral but acquire it from the general environment as we have already discussed.

There are many other examples of populations being contaminated by products discharged into the atmosphere from adjacent factories. A report of raised blood levels of cadmium in residents of a Somerset village in England which had been built on the site of an old zinc mine illustrates this important problem. Zinc and cadmium commonly occur together and reports of discoloured vegetables and of mysterious disorders in cattle grazing locally led to the discovery of abnormally high levels of cadmium in this Somerset village of Shipham[14].

The acute effects of cadmium poisoning, such as respiratory disability from the inhalation of cadmium fumes associated with proliferation of Type II pneumocytes, was not seen in this population. Nor was acute painful skeletal collapse described in areas of zinc mining and smelting in Northern Japan. However, the question of more subtle effects of cadmium intoxication, such as the production of hypertension in the local population, arose.

Blood cadmium levels were raised in two thirds of the residents of Shipham and an increased excretion of 2-microglobulin in their urine suggested that the cadmium was exerting a nephrotoxic effect. There was also an increased prevalence of hypertension. Whilst the nephrotoxicity of cadmium is well established, the cardiotoxic effects are more debatable. Elevation of blood cadmium in untreated hypertensives and the production of hypertension in animals given cadmium support a cardiotoxic effect. This may be produced by the effect of cadmium on the kidney tubules or may be more direct because cadmium displaces divalent cations in enzymes such as monoamine oxidases that inactivate catecholamines.

Smelting of zinc, copper, lead and other metals can also lead to atmospheric pollution by oxides of arsenic because arsenic is often a component of the ores containing these metals. Here again the hazards are not confined to those who work in direct contact with the ores but also affect the surrounding population. The average mortality rates from lung cancer were significantly increased in countries in the USA where metal smelting and refining was going on[15].

Injuries in work places of various sorts are legion. Often they are simple traumatic wounds but occasionally the causative agent may produce multiple effects,

a knowledge of which is essential if proper treatment and prevention of serious incapacity is to be achieved. Injuries from high pressure paint guns illustrate this problem well[16]. High pressure paint guns were first used in the 1950s for the injection of paints, lacquers and the spraying of anti-rust materials on cars. The injuries produced by such guns tend to occur most often in the non-dominant hand and result from the injection of paint materials at high pressure (200–500 kg/cm) into the limb. At first glance these seem to be simple puncture wounds but the spread of the paint material within the limb can cause extensive damage which is so severe as to lead to amputation. Extensive decompression is necessary under general anaesthetic and the use of steroids helps to reduce the inflammatory response.

The solvent rather than the paint itself causes tissue damage. This leads to rapid necrosis with extensive acute inflammatory oedema. Fat and myelin sheaths are dissolved so that the limb becomes locally anaesthetized. Pressure of the extensive exudate, particularly in confined spaces in the hand, obstructs arteries and veins so that arterial spasm and venous thrombosis add to the extent of tissue damage.

High pressure paint spray gun injuries are now well recognized and the important fact that the small pressure entry hole can bear no relation to the subsequent extensive tissue damage is appreciated by orthopaedic surgeons. It is less well known that general toxic effects can result from the injected material such as lead poisoning when lead-containing paint is involved[17].

Industrial poisoning by inorganic compounds of lead such as the sulphate and oxide are hazards that are well known and rarely occur. Organic compounds such as tetraethyl lead in petrol are less well appreciated as dangerous poisons. Cases have been reported in workers cleaning petrol tanks that have contained leaded petrol without due precautions such as the use of masks[18].

Despite the fact that lead poisoning or plumbism has been known for over 100 years it continues to appear as new and unexpected sources arise[19]. For example, the association of Indian eyeliner with lead poisoning has only been recently recognized.

Laboratory workers are exposed to such a wide variety of potentially toxic materials that they might be expected to produce a diversity of disease not encountered in the general population. However, they tend to come from higher socio-economic groups and are more aware than most of the risks of their occupations. Amongst medical laboratory workers infection risks such as tuberculosis and serum hepatitis are recognized. Bladder cancer in those using carcinogenic aromatic amines has been occasionally reported. There is sound experimental evidence to warrant this association. Excess deaths from lymphatic and haemopoietic neoplasms in English male pathologists is not so easily explained particularly as no other neoplasms were notable as compared to the general population[20]. Such neoplasms are often associated with immunodepletion of various sorts and could be due to the effect of some unsuspected environmental agent.

Laboratory workers have often in the past taken undue risks with a variety of chemical substances. This was partly due to the lack of knowledge of their potential danger. Formaldehyde vapour, which is both a primary irritant and a sensitizing agent, is an example. When the odour is detectable the concentration in the atmosphere may have an irritant effect on the eyes and air passages. Concentrations undetectable by smell alone are still potent skin sensitizers, and skin reactions in sensitized persons can be elicited by formaldehyde solutions containing as little as one part in five million of saline[21].

Human beings create hazards whatever they do. Concern about the level of noise in industry, which may be over 90 decibels when one has to shout to be heard, is not matched by concern for the level of noise in discos and the like. Yet noise can not only damage the inner ear as in 'boilermakers' deafness', it can also have more subtle effects such as causing a rise of diastolic pressure which lasts longer than the duration of the sound[22].

Work, play and living in general are hazardous occupations.

Bibliography

1. Cooper, D. K. C. (1971). Accidents in agriculture. *Injury*, **3**, 1
2. Cooper, D. K. C. (1969). Agricultural accidents: a study of 132 patients seen at Addenbrooke's hospital, Cambridge in 12 months. *Br. Med. J.*, **4**, 193
3. Steele-Bodger, A. (1969). Hazards of animal handling. *Ann. Occup. Hyg.*, **12**, 79
4. Wood, W., Gabica, J., Brown, H. W., Watson, M. and Benson, W. W. (1971). Implication of organophosphate pesticide poisoning in the plane crash of a duster pilot. *Aerospace Med.*, **42**, 1111
5. Pesticides turning the corner? (1969). *BIBRA Bull.*, **2**, 499
6. Knight, B. (1977). Hazards of the fishing industry. In Tedeschi, C. G., Eckert, W. G. and Tedeschi, L. G. (eds.), *Forensic Medicine: a Study in Trauma and Environmental Hazards. Vol. III: Environmental Hazards*, p. 1167 (Philadelphia: W. B. Saunders Co.)
7. Leader. (1975). Diving doctors. *Lancet*, **1**, 440
8. Hendry, W. T., Childs, C. M. and Proctor, D. M. (1978). The offshore scene and its hazards. In Mason, J. K. (ed.), *The Pathology of Violent Injury*. (London: Edward Arnold)
9. Soloway, H. B. and Robinson, E. F. (1972). The coagulation mechanism in experimental pulmonary fat embolism. *J. Trauma*, **12**, 630
10. Gresham, G. A. (1975). *A Colour Atlas of Forensic Pathology*. (London: Wolfe)
11. Nicoll, E. A. (1949). Fractures of the dorso-lumbar spine. *J. Bone Jt. Surg. B*, **31**, 376
12. Leader. (1976). Exposure to asbestos dust. *Br. Med. J.*, **1**, 1361
13. Ehrenreich, T. and Selikoff, I. J. (1983). Disease associated with asbestos exposure: diagnostic perspectives in forensic pathology. *Am. J. Forensic Med. Pathol.*, **4**, 63
14. Carruthers, M. and Smith, B. (1979). Evidence of cadmium toxicity in a population living in a zinc mining area. Pilot survey of Shipham residents. *Lancet*, **1**, 845
15. Blot, W. J. and Fraumeni, J. F. Jr. (1975). Arsenical air pollution and lung cancer. *Lancet*, **2**, 142
16. Booth, C. M. (1977). High pressure paint gun injuries. *Br. Med. J.*, **2**, 1333
17. Lilis, R., Green, S. M., Field, J. and Fischbein, A. (1981). Paint spray gun injury of the hand. Report of an unusual source of lead poisoning. *J. Am. Med. Assoc.*, **246**, 1233
18. Beattie, A. D., Moore, M. R. and Goldberg, A. (1972). Tetraethyl-lead poisoning. *Lancet*, **2**, 12
19. Graham, J. A. G., Maxton, D. G. and Twort, C. H. C. (1981). Painters palsy: a difficult case of lead poisoning. *Lancet*, **2**, 1159
20. Harrington, J. M. and Shannon, H. S. (1975). Mortality study of pathologists and medical laboratory technicians. *Br. Med. J.*, **2**, 329
21. Loomis, T. A. (1979). Formaldehyde toxicity. *Arch. Pathol. Lab. Med.*, **103**, 321
22. Leader. (1981). Noise at work. *Br. Med. J.*, **283**, 458

Chapter 5

Injury at Play

All sorts of sporting activity carry some risk: some such as hang-gliding, horse-riding, marathon running, boxing and others carry more risk than many. It would be a sad day if people were deterred from leisure activities by fear of injury. Equally it is important to know the risk and take adequate precautions. Sudden death in men over 40 whilst playing squash racquets is notorious to coroner's pathologists. Sudden death in players of rugby football and referees with a mean age of about 30 years is another well recognized event[1]. Competitive sports are more dangerous because the individual cannot determine his own pace but again joggers can occasionally reduce their blood pressures to zero.

Graduated, carefully selected exercise has an important part to play in the prevention of ischaemic heart disease. It has a number of effects including improved fibrinolytic activity of the blood and so on. The importance of 'warming up' and graduating the exercise to the powers of the individual cannot be emphasized too strongly. Even young athletes in their twenties may die suddenly whilst swimming, rowing or running. The cause is often premature ischaemic heart disease due to narrowing of coronary arteries by atherosclerosis (Figure 5.1). Occasionally only one vessel is severely narrowed with its lumen reduced by 85%. Often there is major narrowing of all three main vessels. Such deaths tend to occur in hyperlipidaemic families particularly in those with Type II hyperlipidaemia. Occasionally as in the lady whose artery is shown in Figure 5.1, no hyperlipidaemia existed. In such rare instances the possibility of some other genetically induced arterial damage must be supposed though its nature remains obscure at present.

Sudden death in young athletes is rarely due to other causes such as atrial septal defect unsuspected in life. Hypertrophic obstructive cardiomyopathy is another cause and rarely evidence of myocarditis may be found. Figure 5.2 illustrates extensive scarring of the subpericardial muscle in a young man who died suddenly after completing 36 lengths of the swimming bath. He had been an active swimmer from the age of 5. Six months before he had suffered a 'dizzy turn' after arduous

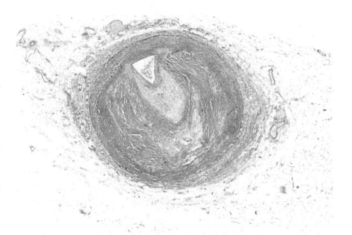

Figure 5.1 *A coronary artery showing a tiny lumen due to progressive deposition of pink atherosclerotic material within the black elastic lamina*

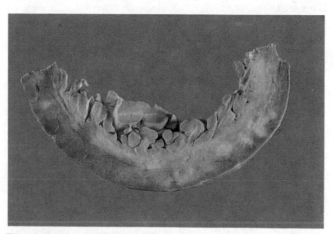

Figure 5.2 *Low power view of a slice of left ventricle showing white fibrous tissue in the outer part of the wall. This distribution of fibrous tissue is more like that of myocarditis than ischaemic fibrosis*

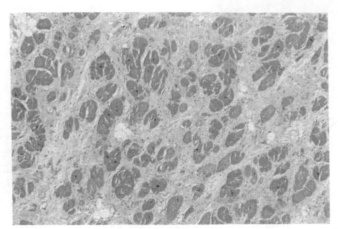

Figure 5.3 *A higher power view of left ventricle in Figure 5.2 showing fibrous tissue around myocardial fibres*

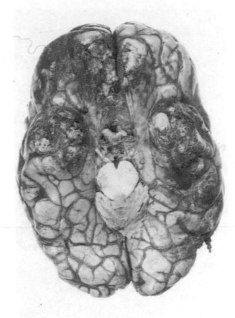

Figure 5.4 *Severe contusion and laceration of the frontal and temporal poles of the brain on their inferior surfaces. This followed a violent blow to the lower jaw. Boxers may suffer milder injuries but the distribution of damage is the same*

swimming. Histological examination of the heart revealed chronic fibrous damage separating individual fibres and evidence also of recent fibre destruction (Figures 5.2, 5.3). A curious feature was the presence of abundant mast cells in the areas of myocardial damage. Examination of his serum revealed no antibodies to Coxsackie or EB viruses nor was there any toxoplasmic antibody. Coxsackie B virus is one of the well-established causes of viral myocarditis in the young. During the active phase of the disease the extent of muscle destruction is related to the amount of exercise taken. Young mice infected with the virus and made to swim in warm water die much more often than infected mice that are not so exercised[2].

The object of this chapter is not to list the numerous injuries that occur in various sorts of sporting activity but rather to indicate special hazards peculiar to particular sports. In so doing it is hoped to create awareness of the special injuries and to enable more care to be taken in their prevention.

Combat

Many games such as rugby football involve personal combat for one reason or another. This section is devoted to those sports where personal combat is the only aim and the overpowering of a contestant is the signal of success. Boxing, wrestling and karate are examples of such activities.

Boxing is still a popular sport and a great deal of controversy exists about its dangers, ways of preventing them and the need to modify the rules of the game. Boxing existed in ancient Crete and no sport was more popular with the ancient Greeks than pugilism. The epics of Homer describe the activities of fist fighters. Prize fighting was popular in England in the early eighteenth century and was a bare-fisted mixture of punching and wrestling. At that time up until the first part of this century there was practically no medical supervision of

boxers. The 'punch drunk' syndrome described in 1928 subsequently became a matter of serious concern and led to proper medical supervision and the elimination of those who were found to have suffered brain damage from the sport.

Minor injuries are commonly seen in boxers. Fracture of the nasal septum and the auricular cartilages followed by haematoma causes the 'cauliflower ear'. Eyebrow lacerations are also frequent and if repeated may end a boxer's career. Maxillary and mandibular fractures are rare and have become much less because of preliminary binding of the boxer's hands, the use of heavier gloves and of gum shields. The hand covering has also reduced the occurrence of metacarpal fractures.

Brain injury is the most serious hazard of boxing. An extensive enquiry by the Royal College of Physicians in 1969 showed clearly that repeated blows to the head will damage its contents. The severity of the damage is directly related to the number of bouts that have been fought[3].

Acute fatal injury may result from subdural haemorrhage. This occurs usually in the middle cranial fossae from tearing of the emissary veins between the dura and the surface of the temporal poles (Figures 5.4–5.6). Several impacts are necessary to produce this lesion consistently. However, a single severe blow to the lower jaw or face as may occur in vehicle injuries can produce the same effect. In such cases there is usually an associated fracture across the base of the skull running through the pituitary fossa (Figure 5.7).

If the boxer survives the subdural haemorrhage becomes adherent to the brain or dura and organizes

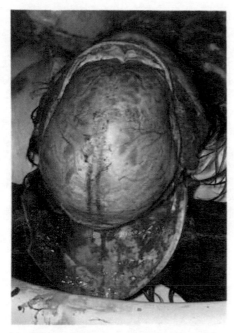

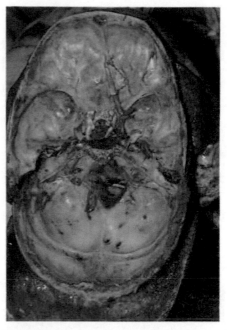

Figure 5.5 *Purple subdural haemorrhage following a blow to the left occipital region indicated by a bruise in the deep scalp*

Figure 5.7 *Transverse fracture across the base of the skull following a severe blow to the face*

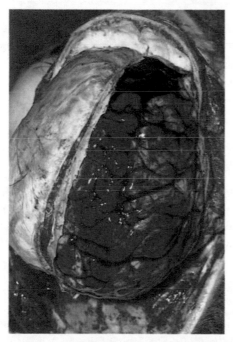

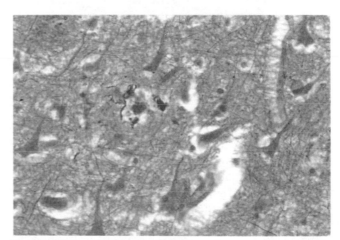

Figure 5.6 *Same case as Figure 5.5 with the dura reflected to show the subdural haemorrhage most conspicuous in the right frontal area. This is the area of 'contrecoup'*

Figure 5.8 *So-called senile plaque in a section of brain stained black by a silver method*

progressively over the next few weeks. Liquefaction may occur within this organized haematoma and the osmotic effects of the small molecules released in the process may cause the membrane to swell with the development of fatal pressure on the brain. Subdural haemorrhage usually requires severe or repeated head injury for its production. In the elderly, however, trivial and even unnoticed injuries may produce such haemorrhages leading to confusion, loss of consciousness and death.

Chronic changes in the brain are included under the heading of traumatic encephalopathy. They include changes in the brain which are similar in some ways to those found in elderly subjects who have never boxed. The clinical features of elderly boxers include progressive dementia, ataxia and features of Parkinsonism. The dementia has been associated with chronic frontal and temporal lesions in one series[4]. The lesions are sunken, haemosiderin-stained areas of the superficial cortex in these areas.

The other clinical features are readily explicable by the chronic lesions that characterize such brains and have been well summarized by Corsellis *et al.*[5] They have identified 'a relatively stereotyped pattern of structural change in the brain'.

They comprise changes in the septum pellucidum, patches of cerebral and cerebellar scarring, loss of the substantia nigra and widespread neurofibrillary tangles

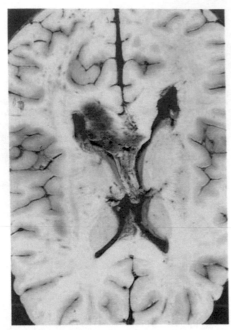

Figure 5.9 *Horizontal slice of brain showing tearing and haemorrhage into the septum pellucidum, the consequence of a shear injury*

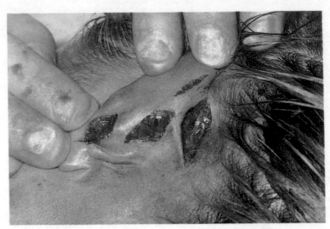

Figure 5.10 *Lacerations behind the ear inflicted with the toe of a shod foot*

in the brain. These are not accompanied by the senile plaques as are found in senile dements from other causes (Figure 5.8). Focal scars are also found in the brains of elderly dements but the occurrence of such lesions in the inferolateral and tonsillar regions of the cerebellum are rare whereas in boxers they are frequent.

Cavitation or rupture of the septum pellucidum is a common feature in the brains of boxers. Such changes are usually traumatic in origin and result from repeated stretching of the thin septum either by direct shearing forces or because of the progressive ventricular enlargement which accompanies the cortical atrophy (Figure 5.9).

Much serious injury in boxing has been eliminated by strict medical supervision and changes in the rules of the sport. It still remains a dangerous sport with the ever-present risk of damage to the brain. It must, however, be kept in proper perspective. Of 1900 head injuries admitted to the neurosurgical unit at Glasgow 52 were due to sport. The sports most commonly associated with head injury were golf, horse-riding and Association football[6]. Another report describes serious chronic brain injury in four National Hunt jockeys[7].

Wrestling does not present the serious injuries that may occur in boxing. The only specific injury associated with this sport is injury to the cervical spinal cord when a bridge is formed by a wrestler. This involves hyperextension of the neck and part of the training of a professional wrestler is to exercise the neck muscles to prevent its occurrence. Damage to the ligaments of the knees and shoulders may occur and lead to chronic disability. This is due to twisting of the limbs.

Interest in the martial arts of self-defence has become

increasingly popular. Karate is a sport that depends upon co-ordination of determination, nerves and muscles. The aim is to release a short burst of powerful energy. Blows are delivered with various parts of both limbs followed by rapid withdrawal[8].

A relatively weak blow can be delivered with the sole of the foot and a much more ferocious kick with the heel. The hand is used in a chopping motion and in other ways. Powerful blows can also be given with knees and elbows. The art of karate demands great self-control and an accurate knowledge of the potential, sometimes lethal, effects of the injuries inflicted. For example, a blow to the neck with the side of the hand can fracture the thyroid cartilages and produce tearing of the carotid arteries.

Indiscriminate kicking as a mode of attack has become increasingly frequent in the United Kingdom. It is now the third most frequent injury in homicidal cases being superseded only by stabbing and manual strangulation. The victim is usually tripped or pushed to the ground. Blows from the toe of the shod foot leave characteristic curved lacerations in concavities of the body such as behind the ears (Figure 5.10), beneath the jaw, side of the neck and so on. Kicking may be followed by stamping on the body leading to bony fractures and extensive bruising[9].

Head injuries in such cases may involve damage to scalp, skull, meninges and brain as seen in any other severe head trauma. A particular injury caused by a blow to the base of the skull deserves mention. This is a rapidly fatal subarachnoid haemorrhage caused by stretching and tearing of the vertebral artery in its course in the first cervical vertebra as it passes into the skull. A fracture of the first vertebral transverse process is sometimes found as well.

Hard contest sport

These sports include Association football, Rugby Union, Rugby League, American football, lacrosse, hockey and so on. Statistics of death and injury are not accurately recorded and accounts are often restricted to individual case reports.

A prospective study of 185 players in 10 British Rugby clubs showed that 53% were injured in a single session[10]. Forwards had more injuries than those who played back and the leg was the most frequent site of injury. Static play and play on wet pitches gave rise to more head and neck injuries but strangely neck injuries were not the result of scrummaging. Body weight, degree of fitness, and degrees of joint mobility bore no relationship to the tendency for injury. Most of the injuries occurred in the latter part of the games and foul play could have been implicated in 31% of them.

There have been other reports suggesting that injuries to the cervical spine occurred rarely in Rugby football. This view is not unanimous, however. Experience in Cardiff has shown that these injuries are becoming more frequent[11]. Dislocation or subluxation of the mid-cervical spine were the predominant lesions in five men who had damage to the spinal cord. The injuries occurred mainly in the scrummage or after a tackle. Four of the patients were irreversibly paralysed. The authors recommend that players should be aware of the hazard of allowing severe flexion forces to be applied to the neck whilst the head is fixed as in a scrum. Collapse of the scrum and deliberate clashing of heads is particularly dangerous for inexperienced players with untrained neck muscles.

Association and Rugby football, like many other hard contest sports, are associated with an array of skeletal injuries. Broken bones, dislocated hand bones, and minor and severe head injuries occur occasionally but are not specific to any of these sports. Association football presents special problems because of the great pressure on professional players to return to the game as soon as is possible after injury.

It is debatable whether repeated trauma to the joints of the lower limbs predispose to osteoarthrosis later in life. However, pubic osteitis and chronic sacroiliac joint disease do seem to be due to twisting of the pelvis brought about by skidding on the field of play[12].

In American football high tackling and the use of charges by the head and shoulders make the game dangerous. Despite the use of helmets, face guards and padding, head injuries are frequent, varying in severity from concussion to cerebral lacerations and extradural haemorrhage from rupture of the middle meningeal artery involved in fracture of the squamous temporal bones. The heavily weighted head can also impose severe strain on the cervical spine with consequent spinal cord damage. This follows a fall after the body has been propelled forward.

Other injuries that occur are less serious but can give rise to chronic disabilty. The knee joint is particularly vulnerable with tearing of the medial and anterior cruciate ligaments or of the medial meniscus. Stretching of trunk and leg muscles leads to muscle rupture and the formation of painful haematomas.

Damage to internal organs is rare in this and other hard contest sports. Kicks in the loin can cause rupture of a kidney. Splenic rupture is rare but the enlarged spleen of infectious mononucleosis is especially vulnerable and emphasizes the importance of temporarily excluding persons with any sort of suspected viral infection from such activity.

A number of other ball games are surprisingly free from a record of serious injuries. Squash racquets has proliferated as a popular game in the United Kingdom over recent years. It demands bursts of severe physical effort from the players but injury is rare. Even injuries to the ball of the eye are rare. The squash ball is of such a size as to fit into the orbit and of all the 'bat and ball' games squash provides more eye injuries than the rest, but they are rare[13].

More dangerous than these minor injuries is the effect of the exercise cult that has brought many middle-aged coronary-prone individuals into the exercise scene. There is a widespread notion that exercise is a good thing because it rejuvenates, prevents heart attacks, increases libido and leads to endorphin release in the brain. This cult has been associated with reports of sudden death in squash players, marathon runners and so on. This raises the opposing question: is exercise bad for the heart and does a pathological state of athlete's heart exist? All forms of exercise will increase cardiac output. The trained athlete has a high exercise stroke volume of the heart which maintains a high exercise output and achieves maximum lung perfusion on exercise. The stroke volume can be increased by enlargement of the left ventricle or by more efficient systolic emptying of the chambers. This means that the ejection fraction remaining in diastole is reduced. This ejection fraction is about 60–75% and is the same in trained and untrained people. The efficiency of the heart of the trained athlete is due to increased size of the left ventricle. Because it is bigger it beats more slowly at rest and still maintains an adequate output. The cause of 'athlete's bradycardia' is more an intrinsic quality of the large heart rather than an effect of increased vagal tone ('after all an elephant's heart beats more slowly than that of a mouse'[14]).

The modern view is that enlargement of the athlete's heart is a physiological response to repeated exercise. Nevertheless, sudden death does occur following severe exercise and the majority of these cases have a cardiac cause which we have already discussed. Lesions in the cardiovascular system may be obvious such as anomalous origin of the left coronary artery, coronary atheroma, myocarditis or aortic rupture. Occasionally lesions are not found. This is most often due to failure to examine the heart thoroughly. No examination of such cases is complete without a study of the conducting system. It is now known that 0.1% of the population has major defects of the conducting mechanism in the heart. The Wolff–Parkinson–White anomaly is an example. Such persons are liable to drop dead suddenly without revealing any obvious cause at post-mortem examination.

Sports not involving hard contest

New types of sporting activity are constantly appearing. Skateboard riding and hang-gliding are examples. Old sports are also being revived, a popular example being the marathon race. It was introduced as a road race at the revival of the Olympic games at Athens in 1896. It was based on the legend of the Greek soldier who ran 22 miles from Marathon to Athens to recount the victory of Greeks over the Persians.

The London marathon of 1982 was run over a distance of 26 miles, there being some 60 000 applicants wishing to participate. Most of the race is done on roads and pavements and results in repetitive jarring injuries to the legs. It is not surprising that the bulk of damage occurs at the knee joint or below it. This is despite the construction of pliable, compressible footwear designed to minimize the injury.

Damage to the Achilles tendon is a common form of marathon injury. This may take the form of an acute inflammation of the tendon sheath or even rupture of the tendon itself. Shin splints is the name given to pain in the front of the leg following protracted exercise. It is due to swelling of the anterior tibial muscles in the tight anterior compartment of the leg. The cause of the swelling is not clear but imbalance between the strong calf muscles and the weaker anterior tibial has been suggested as a factor[15].

Stress fractures of the fibula and tibia are also found in marathon runners and in joggers. The term shin splints is often applied to these fractures rather than to the syndrome of the anterior tibial compartment. Such fractures are often not visible radiologically until two or more weeks after the fracture. The radiological appearance that develops is one of subperiosteal new bone formation and may mimic changes due to syphilis, osteogenic sarcoma or healed rickets. The changes are probably due to the severe pulling on tendinous attachments giving rise to underlying minor infractions of bone. If the runner is slightly knock-kneed or bow-legged the imbalance of the foot may predispose to abrasion of the articular surface of the patella on the lower femoral condyles. This results in chondromalacia of the patella and may predispose to subsequent osteoarthrosis. Avascular necrosis of the tibial tuberosity (Osgood–Schlatter disease) is another possible complication of long-distance running in young people.

The major cause of 'collapse' in the London marathon of 1982 was dehydration and long-distance runners are well advised to ensure an adequate intake of fluid during exercise. This dehydration can lead to intravascular clumping of red cells and platelets. In one case a 14-year-old school boy developed dysphasia and a right hemiplegia after running 10 miles through the streets of Dublin. He recovered completely which probably indicated a temporary middle cerebral artery blockage due to platelets which subsequently lysed.

Running has been described as a 'positive addiction' for regular adherents and inability to do so may lead to a withdrawal syndrome[16]. Some psychiatrists have described running as more successful therapy for mild depression than psychotherapy. Others have treated anxiety, anorexia, schizophrenia and phobias by prescribing running. The drive to run is illustrated by those who developed myocardial infarction despite warning symptoms which they ignored when running.

Coronary artery occlusion may follow violent exertion although not all authors would agree with this. Some report unusual exertion in only 2% preceding the attack but other series indicate that vigorous activity may precede the infarction in 22% of subjects[17]. The danger increases with the age of the individual. Considerable caution must be exercised before accepting jogging and other exercise as a usual prophylactic for coronary artery disease in the middle aged.

In recent years a variety of devices have been produced to enable sporting activities on land, sea and in the air. They are interesting because they illustrate patterns of injury that relate to the method of transport. A study of these injuries should enable the maximum design to ensure safety. A few examples will be studied to illustrate this point.

The invention of the skateboard has led to a few minor and sometimes major injuries. Most of the damage is to the forearms. Occasionally, skull fractures, concussion, splenic rupture and retroperitoneal haemorrhage due to deceleration occur. Helmets and protective pads on the limbs do not help to prevent these injuries. The provision of designated areas for skateboarding seems to be the only practical way of reducing casualties from this sport[18].

Surprisingly little has been written about injuries caused by playground equipment. A recent report of 200 children injured by playground equipment indicated that 26.5% had fractures. The more severe injuries seem to be associated with slides and climbing frames rather than with swings and other equipment.

Injury incurred at speed

There is no limit to the ways in which people amuse themselves by travelling at speed on land, water and in the air. Various sorts of vehicles are used, the car, motor cycle and horse being the oldest established. New methods such as hang-gliding, water-skiing and the like constantly arise. Injuries sustained at speed are a combination of direct trauma and the serious effects of indirect injury caused by rapid deceleration of the body on collision. These injuries are caused by continued movement of organs when movement of the body as a whole ceases. As a result various structures such as the heart, lungs, gut and kidney break loose from their attachments. Similar injuries occur in accidents during travel by land and air. The compulsory use of seat belts in cars in the UK has had a significant effect in reducing some of these injuries.

Lack of proper instruction is one of the main causes of trouble in newly developed sporting activities. Hang-gliding is a good example of this. The British Hang-Gliding Association accident report records only two deaths in 1975[19]. The majority of injuries was limb fractures due to high wind speed, turbulence and stalling but inexperience was the main factor[19]. The apparatus is a V-shaped set of aluminium tubes made rigid with wires and carrying about 18.5 m² of sail. The pilot is suspended beneath this in a seat with an A-shaped frame which he grips. By shifting forwards or sideways in his seat he can direct the machine. In such an exposed situation the pilot is clearly vulnerable to a variety of features if things go wrong. There are about 6000 hang-gliders in Britain and the risk of injury is about the same as that of riding a motorcycle. However, the number of reported injuries is probably less than actually occur partly because staff in accident departments regard the sport with ridicule[20].

Reports from the Austrian Tyrol take a more serious view of the dangers of hang-gliding and recommend a number of precautions to be taken before embarking on this activity[21]. The authors, like others, emphasize the important role of experience and training in the sport.

Parachuting is another popular aerial activity and injuries are not frequent. They can occur on exit from the aircraft, from failures of parachute development and on landing. Landing is the most hazardous part of the activity and can result in limb fractures and compression fractures of the pelvis and spine. Deceleration injuries to the spleen, liver, lungs, heart and thoracic aorta rarely occur. Only very rarely is pre-existing disease like myocardial infarction a factor in parachute accidents. Descents from unacceptably high altitudes may result in hypoxia and loss of control. Descents should not be made from altitudes in excess of 4600 m.

Human inventiveness precludes any chapter on sporting activities from being complete. Careful documentation of any accidents that may occur is essential in order to ascertain patterns of injury that will enable suitable precautions to be taken. Examples of this sort of problem are numerous.

Water-skiing injuries by boat propellers can largely be prevented by the use of tow ropes of appropriate length. Vaginal and rectal injuries due to water douch-ing are avoided by wearing tight rubber pants when skiing.

The therapeutic advantages of all sorts of sporting activities are considerable. This chapter is not intended to diminish enthusiasm but to advise caution and proper precautions against serious injury. When Winston Churchill had been knocked down by a taxi in America he said 'Live dangerously, take things as they come, dread nought, all will be well.'

Bibliography

1. Opie, L. H. (1975). Sudden death and sport. *Lancet*, **1**, 263
2. Grist, N. R. and Bell, E. J. (1969). Coxsackie viruses and the heart. *Am. Heart J.*, **77**, 295
3. Leader. (1973). Boxing brains. *Lancet*, **2**, 1065
4. Johnson, J. (1960). Neuropathology of boxing, *Br. J. Psychiat.*, **115**, 45
5. Corsellis, J. A. N., Brunton, C. J. and Freeman-Browne, D. (1973). The aftermath of boxing. *Psychol. Med.*, **3**, 270
6. Lindsay, K. W., McLatchie, G. and Jennet, B. (1980). Serious head injury in sport. *Br. Med. J.*, **281**, 789
7. Foster, J. B., Leiguarda, R. and Tilley, P. J. B. (1976). Brain damage in National Hunt jockeys. *Lancet*, **1**, 981
8. Watson, A. J. (1978). Kicking, karate and kung fu. In Mason, J. K. (ed.), *The Pathology of Violent Injury*. (London: Edward Arnold)
9. Teare, R. D. (1961). Blows with the shod foot. *Med. Sci. Law*, **1**, 429
10. Davies, J. E. and Gibson, T. (1978). Injuries in Rugby Union football. *Br. Med. J.*, **2**, 1759
11. Williams, J. P. R. and McKibbin, B. (1978). Cervical spine injuries in Rugby football. *Br. Med. J.*, **2**, 1747
12. Harris, N. H. and Murray, R. O. (1974). Lesions of the symphysis in athletes. *Br. Med. J.*, **4**, 211
13. Barrell, G. V., Cooper, P. J., Elkington, A. R., Macfadyen, J. M., Powel, R. G. and Tormey, P. (1983). Squash ball to eye ball. The likelihood of squash players incurring an eye injury. *Br. Med. J.*, **283**, 893
14. Pedoe, D. T. (1983). Sports injuries. Cardiological problems. *Br. J. Hosp. Med.*, **29**, 213
15. Temple, C. (1983). Sports injuries. Hazards of jogging and marathon running. *Br. J. Hosp. Med.*, **29**, 237
16. Colt, E. W. D. and Spyropoulos, E. (1976). Running and stress fractures. *Br. Med. J.*, **2**, 706
17. Black, A., Black, M. M. and Gensini, G. (1975). Exertion and coronary artery injury. *Angiology*, **26**, 759
18. Illingworth, C., Jay, A., Parkin, R., Collic, M., Noble, D., Robson, V. and Isley, A. (1977). Skateboard injuries: preliminary report. *Br. Med. J.*, **2**, 1636
19. Yuill, G. M. (1977). Icarus's syndrome: new hazards in flight. *Br. Med. J.*, **1**, 823
20. Leader. (1978). Hazards of hang gliding. *Br. Med. J.*, **1**, 388
21. Margreiter, R. and Lugger, L. J. (1978). Hang gliding accidents. *Br. Med. J.*, **1**, 400

Chapter 6

Injury at Home

Serious accidents in the home are remarkably infrequent considering the wide range of hazards that exist in the average home. Many home injuries affect the young and the very old and are often due to lack of forethought and the proper maintenance of equipment. The home is also a closed sequestered environment within which all sorts of acts can be perpetrated. Abuse of children and others is an increasingly common activity that can go undetected. The abuse varies from obvious physical violence to more subtle psychological injury that is often difficult to verify.

Accidental injury is one of the world's modern epidemics. Accidents are the commonest single cause of death in young children and also result in much disability[1]. Younger children are at greater risk than older ones but all are vulnerable. It is a sad affair that dangerous situations in the home are often not recognized until a calamity has occurred. Figure 6.1 shows a 2-year-old child that hung herself accidently on the torn hem of a curtain. She had been allowed to play by twisting herself in the curtain until the lethal noose developed.

Sudden unexpected death in infancy (cot death, crib death) includes a small proportion that are due to either accident or homicide and we shall deal with this matter shortly. Other accidents are often due to faulty design and construction of buildings. Roof gardens and balconies in blocks of flats are special hazards that require fortification against childhood accidents. Secure window fastenings and provision of catches that prevent children opening them to the full can prevent dangerous falls.

The very old, who are often ataxic, deaf and partially sighted, like children are often victims of the home environment. They fall over objects left about the floor, slip on loose bits of carpet, knock over pans and kettles producing fractures, burns and scalds which can be lethal. The very young and the very old are also susceptible to changes of environmental temperature. The

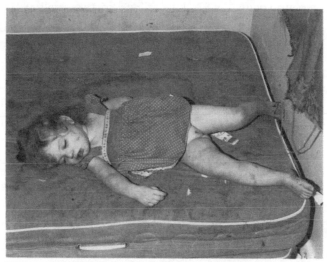

Figure 6.1 *Torn loop of a curtain with which a 5-year-old girl strangled herself. Note ligature mark on neck*

young have a large surface area in relation to volume and lose heat readily under cold conditions. The elderly tend to have lower body temperatures than younger people and hence cool more rapidly to dangerously low temperature levels[2].

Accidental hypothermia in old people was thought to be rare before 1958. The severe winter of 1963 led the Royal College of Physicians to investigate the problem. They defined hypothermia as a rectal temperature below 35 °C (85 °F). Temperatures taken in the mouth are of little value in determining hypothermia because the mouth temperature does not reflect well the 'core' temperature of the body. Rectal readings are not popular so a reliable device for measuring urine temperature was devised[3].

The mortality of hypothermia is about 70% when the core temperature is less than 30 °C and is 32% at core temperatures between 30 °C and 35 °C. The symptoms are insidious and once established hypothermia produces a multitude of confusing clinical features. The patient will not complain of being cold: the reduced alertness prevents this. A variety of focal neurological signs such as focal paralyses, dysarthria and ataxia may develop. Frank shivering is replaced by increased muscle tone with a fine tremor that can be confused with Parkinsonism. The subcutaneous tissues feel firm and cold and the skin often shows blotchy erythema. Bradycardia will be followed by a variety of dysrhythmias culminating in ventricular fibrillation[4]. Respiration is slow and usually accompanied by bronchopneumonia.

Post-mortem findings are often inconclusive. Bronchopneumonia of itself is a not unexpected finding in the elderly. The findings of blotchy cutaneous erythema, ulcers in the stomach, small and large bowel, are suggestive. These ulcers are probably due to haemoconcentration leading to sludging in the microcirculation of the gut. Focal pancreatitis may be due to reflux associated with cold-induced ileus of the small gut. Foci of necrosis may also be found in the liver and myocardium due to microcirculatory obstructions by sludging or spasm. Catecholamine blood levels are raised in these subjects and myocytolytic foci in the heart might be the result of this (Figure 3.49). Similar foci seen in acute intracranial disease and injury are usually attributed to focal vascular spasm in the heart brought about by catecholamine excess. Similar lesions have been produced in rats by injecting sympathomimetic substances such as isoproterenol[5].

In general all the tissues appear red due to the increased binding of oxygen by haemoglobin at low temperatures. A variety of factors such as poverty, alcohol, drugs and senile dementia contribute to accidental hypothermia. Awareness of the possibility by medical and social workers is an important prophylactic.

Dangerous apparatus in the home

Practically every household appliance is capable of inflicting injury. Electrical and heating devices are especially culpable. Incorrect wiring of electrical devices, the insertion of inappropriate fuses, the perforation of cables by nails and screws all contribute to the hazards.

Electrical injuries as a cause of death can prove difficult to detect at autopsy. When death is due to high voltages such as lightning strikes or collapse of overhead power cables (Figure 6.2) burn marks are readily seen. They consist of drying, cracking and lifting of the skin with a peripheral band of erythema. Lower voltages in domestic use may produce no visible lesions if the contact is of short duration. However, faint burns that are suspected of being electrical in origin can be identified as such by the appearance of metals such as copper, aluminium and iron on the lesion using an electrographic method[6].

Because of the paucity of findings in electrical deaths at low voltages it is important to have a high index of

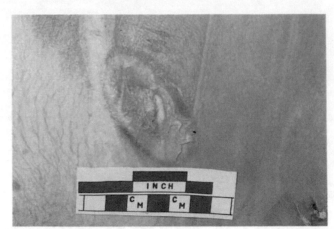

Figure 6.2 *An electrical burn from contact with a collapsed overhead cable. Note the explosive lifting of the skin and the peripheral halo of vasodilatation*

suspicion that electrocution might have occurred. The autopsy may show cardiac dilatation, occasional features of asphyxia such as petechial haemorrhages but little else. However, the circumstances of the death may provide an indication of electrocution. A sudden scream or shout followed by death is a feature and is rare in other forms of death. It often occurs with low voltage electrocution. Another useful feature is the early onset of rigor mortis particularly if it affects an arm or a leg singly. Electrical tetany accelerates the development of rigor mortis.

Detailed examination of the electrical device responsible for the death is clearly important. Incorrect wiring of plugs, short circuits in damaged and old cables, and defects in the appliance itself are common causes of electrocution[7]. If during electrocution another part of the body comes into contact with other metal objects they may leave an impression on the skin surface which may be confusing. A man electrocuted himself with a defective electrical coffee pot, fell to the ground and his head came into contact with a nickel-plated metal grill which left multiple small black burns on the scalp which raised the possibility of wounds due to buck shot[8].

Electrical faults are not infrequently the cause of fires in the home. Decrepit poorly maintained wiring is a feature and television sets are a notable hazard in this respect. Coal fires, gas fires and cookers, electrical fires and cookers and inflammable liquids are all potential sources of conflagration. Serious burns in the home tend to involve the young and the very old. The use of adequate fire guards is essential for both age groups. All too often they succeed in accidentally igniting clothing even though great legislative efforts have been made to try to introduce non-inflammable garments. Most of the deaths from ignition of clothing occur in the elderly. Figure 6.3 indicates the problem. An old lady smoked a cigarette at the same time as using an inflammable hair lacquer. She was unable to move because of a previous stroke. Under such circumstances the body is often almost totally consumed by fire and limbs may

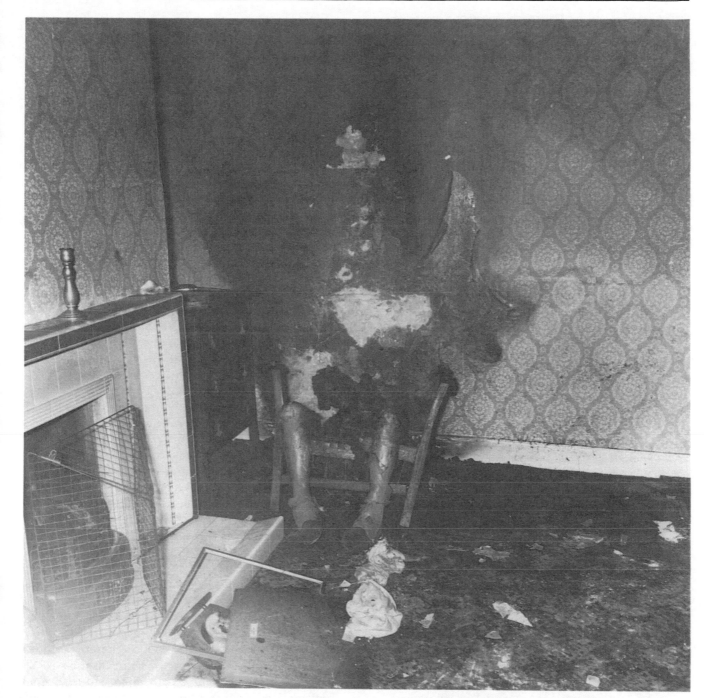

Figure 6.3 *Remains of an old lady consumed by fire. The upper part of the body was totally destroyed*

survive because they drop off the burned body. Deaths in fires present problems because of the chaos and destruction of the environment (Figure 6.4).

Even when the clothing is totally consumed and the entire torso charred it is often possible to find well-preserved internal organs that help in identification of age and sex and may provide a natural cause for collapse that precipitated the cause of the fire. Toxicological analysis may reveal alcohol and other drugs which have played a part in the death.

Post-mortem findings which indicate that death occurred during the fire include carboxyhaemoglobinaemia, soot in the large and small air passages and loss and fraying of tracheal epithelium. This is not always so. Sometimes carboxyhaemoglobulin is not found and soot is present only in the trachea and main bronchi (Figure 6.5). This tends to be the case when fires are accompanied by an explosion which leads to sudden cardiac and respiratory arrest[9]. In those who survive, methaemoglobulinaemia may be found due to the inhalation of oxides or nitrogen derived from burning plastics. Problems that arise in burned survivors are well documented including fluid loss, infection and scarring. Less often there is chronic damage to the air passages. Tracheal stenosis, bronchiectasis and bronchiolitis obliterans have been reported[10].

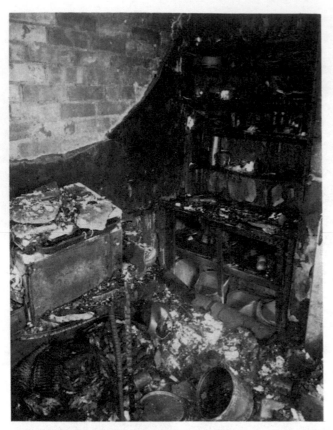

Figure 6.4 *Destructive effects of fire in a small kitchen. Sifting through such debris for human and other remains is a time-consuming business*

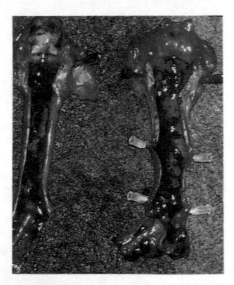

Figure 6.5 *Opened tracheas of two victims of a fire showing soot in both of them*

More subtle effects may result from fires in the home and other confined spaces. These are largely due to carbon monoxide poisoning. The gas is generated whenever a carbonaceous fuel is burned in a space where the oxygen supply is restricted. Coal gas poisoning is now a rare event in the United Kingdom following its replacement by natural gas as a fuel. However, paraffin

heaters and lamps, coal, coke and wood fires can all generate carbon monoxide if ventilation is inadequate. Old people are especially vulnerable because they tend to exclude draughts and other sources of air in order to conserve heat in winter time. Such deaths have occurred in tightly sealed caravans where paraffin lamps are used as a light source, for example. Gas water heaters in small bathrooms continue to be a hazard. This is particularly so when the air vent to the heater is blocked either by a bird's nest or is caused by an unfavourable change of wind direction which prevents the exit of products of combustion. Inadequate ventilation of gas heaters can often be suspected from the gas burning with a yellowish flare and from deposits of carbon on the edge of the burner on the front of the appliance (Figure 6.6). Adequate ventilation is also important when large quantities of natural gas are burned in central heating devices. Regular inspections and servicing should totally prevent such calamities but there are still examples of whole families being overcome by carbon monoxide in houses where equipment is tampered with or inadequately maintained (Figures 6.7, 6.8).

Small animals and children are especially susceptible to carbon monoxide poisoning. This is especially important because of the vulnerability of the child's brain to the poison and can lead to serious, disabling neurological deficits[11] (Figure 6.9). Carbon monoxide poisoning can produce a host of confusing clinical features that may delay accurate diagnosis in the early stages. A family of six suffered from episodic outbreaks of confusion and ataxia. The astute general practitioner observed that the cat and a baby suffered most severely and occasionally lapsed into semi-consciousness. The grandparent of the family was relatively unaffected in these episodes. The cause of the family's problems was ultimately traced to defective combustion in a gas central heating appliance which periodically generated carbon monoxide due to partial obstruction of the duct leading from the heater to the outside air.

Fires in the home can lead to the generation of toxic gases of all sorts. These are a hazard not only to the inhabitants but also to those called upon to deal with a conflagration. The thermal degradation of polyvinyl chloride, a plastic polymer, is particularly important in this regard. Polymers of this sort have been widely used in home construction, furnishings and in covering electrical cables. It is a hard-wearing material which is easy to clean, hence its use. It is not readily inflammable but heat degrades it. Between 225 and 475 °C polyvinyl chloride (PVC) loses 60% of its weight due to the production of hydrogen chloride, chlorine and phosgene, all of which are deadly poisonous gases[12].

The toxicity of phosgene and the other decomposition products of PVC, which include benzene, toluene, xylene, napthalene and vinyl chloride, is small compared to that of hydrogen chloride. This and carbon monoxide are the main toxic hazards of the decomposition of PVC.

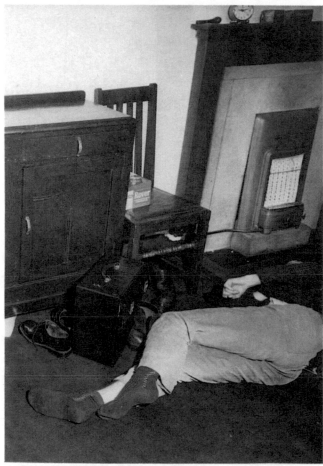

Figure 6.6 *Staining of the upper surround of a gas fire due to imperfect combustion caused by a blockage of the flue*

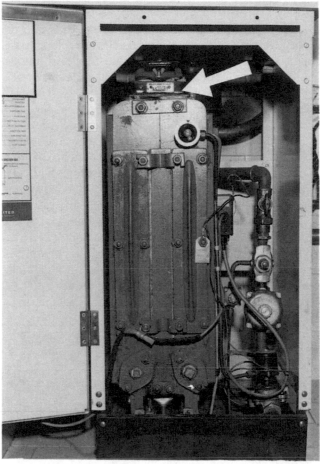

Figure 6.7 *A gas water heater showing the site of a leaking washer on the vent which enabled toxic exhaust gases to escape*

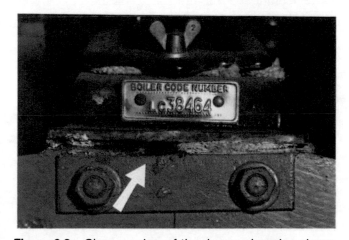

Figure 6.8 *Close up view of the damaged washer shown in Figure 6.7*

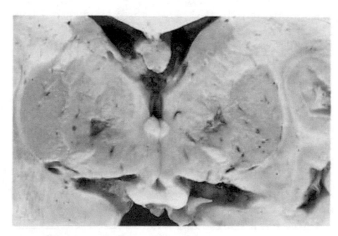

Figure 6.9 *Bilateral symmetrical necrosis of the basal ganglia as is seen after recovery from carbon monoxide poisoning*

Hydrogen chloride is inhaled either as a gas or as hydrochloric acid in water vapour and is a powerful irritant to the mucous membranes of the eyes and of the respiratory tract. 50–100 parts/10^6 are tolerable to human beings for an hour but concentrations higher than that induce laryngeal spasm and pulmonary oedema.

There are two components of smoke: small particles of carbon coated with organic acids and aldehydes and a gaseous fraction. The bulk of this is carbon monoxide and carbon dioxide but a small proportion of other gases is present. These are pulmonary irritants and vary in composition according to the nature of the combusted material. Many such irritants which include nitrogen dioxide, chlorine, sulphur dioxide and ammonia evade the filter trap of the respiratory mucosa and enter the alveoli where they dissolve in water to produce histotoxic acids or alkalis. This leads to a violent inflammatory response with destruction of lung tissue.

Total destruction of bodies can occur in fires particularly in the home. We have already discussed the postmortem examination of bodies found under such conditions but it is well to dwell a little on the dental identification of victims of fire. In homes, vehicular and aircraft accidents teeth may be the only remains for the identification of burned bodies[13].

Cremation of human bodies provides a useful baseline against which to compare the effects of accidental burning on human dental remains. Cremation of human bodies usually consists of incineration at 980 °C for about 1½–2 h. All but dental gold and cobalt steel appliances are destroyed by this process and some distortion of the metals is usually observed.

A two-storey house in Mimico, Ontario was allowed to burn unimpeded as an experiment. It was found that 42 min were needed before the main floor reached 1274 °C; during this time the second floor temperature did not rise above 232 °C. When the ceiling of the main floor collapsed the temperature on the second floor rose to 1004 °C but had dropped to 870 °C 3 min later.

One of the commonest causes of accidental fires in the home is smoking. This may occur in a chair when the occupant falls asleep, often under the influence of alcohol or may occur in bed. Under such circumstances the ignited furniture smoulders for some time and the carbon monoxide produced is often lethal. A sudden rush of air from opening a door or breaking of a window produces a fire of high heat intensity. The temperature achieved is much higher than that achieved in a crematorium and if unchecked leads to total incineration of the body. However, apart from some charring of the anterior incisors the posterior dentition is often unimpaired. This is due to the protection afforded by the moist tongue and the thick facial muscles which contract firmly over the face in the intense heat (Figure 6.10).

Some idea of the temperature and intensity of the fire can be gained from the subsequent state of the dentition. In a car fire in which husband and wife were totally

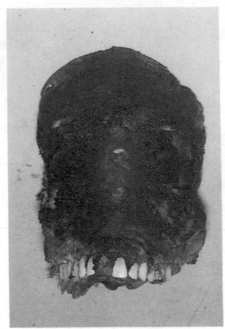

Figure 6.10 *Despite severe burning of the exterior of the body the teeth are often well preserved enabling identification to be done*

incinerated such evidence was available. The wife had two fixed bridges replacing upper second bicuspids and five other gold crowns according to pre-mortem dental records. All of these had melted into a lump of gold. The husband was recorded as having an upper lateral incisor replaced by porcelain fused to a gold restoration with the lateral cantilevered to the central incisor. The porcelain had melted but the gold bridge had kept its form. Dental gold melts at 1024 °C but special gold fused to porcelain melts at 1221 °C. This suggests that the temperature of the fire was in the range of 1024–1221 °C.

Silver amalgam is 72% silver with tin, copper and zinc triturated with mercury. This melts readily and a variety of products of silver, tin, copper and zinc result. Temperatures between 500 °C and 1000 °C cause the amalgam to disintegrate.

Dental prostheses on the whole survive heat poorly: it depends upon the materials from which they are made. Acrylic dentures melt and ignite at 200–250 °C but gold or chrome steel alloys survive much better up to 1100 °C. However, the tongue and facial muscles provide some protection from heat as with a normal dentition.

Dental pulp is another identifiable tissue that can survive intense heat. The dentinal tubules contain 8–10% water. Heating causes the fluid to boil with explosion of the enamel cap. The dentine loses water and shrinks but the original tooth and pulpal form remains enabling some radiographic comparison to be made with pre-mortem dental radiographs.

A good deal can be learned from the dentition of burned bodies. Not only does a study aid identification but it can also provide some idea about the intensity of

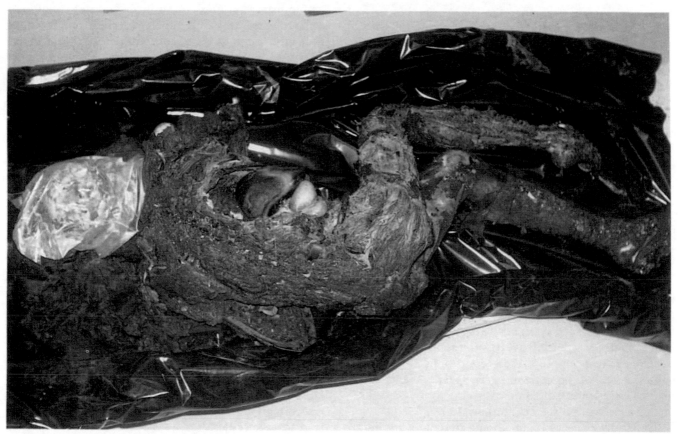

Figure 6.11 *A burned corpse. The intestines and liver have protruded from the burned abdomen but are, like other internal organs, often well preserved*

heat and the duration of a fire. Preservation of dental evidence at a scene of burning is often difficult. The entire scene is usually one of chaos with burned clothes, furniture, flesh, smoke, fumes and unstable floors complicating the situation (Figure 6.11). The assistance of a forensic odontologist under such circumstances is invaluable. Unfortunately in the UK such experts are scarce but it must not be forgotten that the average dental surgeon has a lot to offer in such circumstances.

Radiology of burned bodies is of considerable value, particularly when a number of individuals are thought to have been involved. This is particularly applicable to aircraft accidents. Radiology can help to identify the number of individuals who have been burned and can help to identify foreign materials, not the least bullets, that may be present in and around the body[14].

It is important to remember that burned victims wherever found may not have died as a result of the fire. Circumstances may indicate the need to search for common poisons and a detailed examination of the remains, though a formidable task at first sight, must be made to exclude the possibility of injury unconnected with the burning. Carbon monoxide poisoning is probably not the cause of death when carboxyhaemoglobin concentrations are less than 40%[15].

Burns provide a common cause of morbidity and mortality. About two million people are burned in the United States every year and about 10000 of them die. Most of the deaths are due to burning by fire but the most frequent cause of all burns is contact with hot liquids. Again in the USA about 112000 people are seen with scalds and 2600 of these are caused by hot tap water. The hot water tap is a dangerous appliance particularly to children less than 5 years old, the elderly more than 65 years old and the physically and mentally handicapped. A simple remedy is to set water heaters to a lower temperature. Most electric heaters are preset at 65.5 °C and gas heaters at 60 °C. At these temperatures full thickness epidermal burns may occur in adults after only 2–5 s exposure[16]. It is important to consider legislation to reduce hot water temperatures. Not only will this reduce morbidity but will greatly save energy costs. For example, the lowering of hot water temperature by 10% would save the United States the equivalent cost of 88000 barrels of oil a day.

Immersion in water whether hot or cold can be a source of fatal injury in the home. The hazards of home swimming pools and bathtubs as a cause of drowning in small children have been well emphasized[17]. About 23% of immersion accidents in the Australian Capital Territory were in swimming pools or bathtubs. Less emphasis has been laid on immersion in pails of water. This sort of accident tends to involve children about 10–12 months of age who are usually the youngest in a

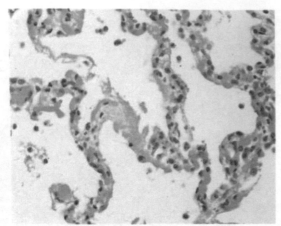

Figure 6.12 *Section of lung from a case of paraquat poisoning showing thickening of interalveolar septa leading to impaired gas perfusion and hypoxia*

large family. The typical family is usually poor, the mother stressed and the child unsupervised at the time of the accident. The contents of the buckets are often contaminated with disinfectant, detergent, ammonia or other cleansing fluid and these contribute to the fatal consequence of immersion. Laryngeal oedema and necrosis is a feature of some cases due to the presence of these irritant substances in the water[18].

Practically every room in a home contains some dangerous items. The bathroom houses a number of lethal objects such as the bathtub, the medicine chest, and water heating devices that may cause electrocution or asphyxia from carbon monoxide produced by combustion of natural gas in a poorly ventilated area.

Outhouses such as garden sheds and garages contain an abundance of hazards. Inflammable liquids such as petrol and paraffin are often poorly labelled and secured. Pesticides with detached labels can be a potent source of poisoning (Figure 6.12). Electrical tools of various sorts are dangerous either because of inadequate guards on them or imperfect wiring and earthing. New tools are being developed regularly and assume common use. The chain saw is such an example. It is now widely used for wood cutting and can injure in various ways. Kickback injuries are not infrequent. The chain saw is responsible for more than 20% of logging accidents[19]. It is a hand-held saw designed for use with the right hand whilst the left hand steadies it. The teeth move forwards on a chain. If the tooth strikes a hard object such as a piece of metal or a knot of wood the saw flies backwards into the face of the operator. This produces an oblique linear laceration but fortunately the eye is rarely injured.

Every power tool has its own particular patterns of injury. Foot lacerations and amputation of toes are a feature of powered lawn mowers. Power planes and saws cause finger and finger pulp amputations and we have already discussed the dire effects of high pressure paint guns.

Abnormal use of objects in and around the home can

lead to bizarre injuries. A variety of household objects such as glue pots and tumblers have been reported after insertion into the rectum for sexual gratification. Insertion of the penis into dustette vacuum cleaners has caused severe lacerations to the glans because the rotating blades of the cleaner are situated 15 cm from the orifice of the suction tube[20].

Economic circumstances sometimes determine the abnormal use of pieces of equipment. During the Great Depression of the 1930s poor families used discarded car battery casing as a convenient source of fuel. This resulted in contamination of the home environment with lead and children developed encephalopathy which occasionally progressed to permanent brain damage[21].

Most homes have step ladders and these are perfectly safe if properly used. If they are improperly placed or poorly maintained they can cause injury. Falls from ladders are not uncommon either to the occupant of the home or to those who clean windows. A variety of orthopaedic injuries occur, notably crush fractures of vertebrae and the calcaneum. Proper securing of ladders and the use of safety belts go far to prevent many of the injuries. The 'rush job' is the dangerous one. Here the height to be reached is not great and the task is seemingly a trivial one of short duration. These factors lead to carelessness[22].

Dangers from animals in the home

Risks from animals are often due to the owner's neglect of the animal. The advantages of household pets such as dogs and cats do not need to be outlined here but ignorance and lack of consideration of the animal by the owner can lead to problems.

One is often amazed at the kinds of animals kept as pets. Monkeys, spiders, snakes, rodents are but a few of the unexpected inhabitants of the home.

Hazards from animals fall into three main groups: traumatic, infective and poisonous. Most of the trauma associated with animals is due to biting and about 90% are attributed to dogs. The wounds tend to occur on the extremities but in young children bites of the face and neck are more common. A study in Jefferson County, Alabama[23] showed the largest number of bites occurred in spring or early summer. About 37% were attributed to specific breeds and about half were German shepherd dogs. Big dogs (more than 23 kg in weight) were more culpable than smaller ones.

Dog bites provide the majority of animal bites. Only 12% of bites were caused by other animals and of these nearly half were caused by cats. The rest were attributed to wild or pet rodents. Only 4% were due to wild animals such as foxes, skunk, raccoon and bats. This small proportion is the only group considered to be important in rabies transmission in the USA.

The old and the young can trip over animals in the home and sustain a variety of injuries. More subtle trauma due to animals is very rare. Young babies can sometimes be overlain by cats whilst in their prams and asphyxial death may occur[24]. Authors in texts of child care are well aware of the problem and advocate the use of cat nets to prevent the animals climbing into a cot or pram. It is surprising that smothering deaths of this sort are not reported more often. Perhaps they are undetected. In such cases the death may be attributed to sudden unexpected death in infancy if the animal has left the cot or pram. If the child survives and subsequently succumbs from hypoxic brain damage it may be labelled as infantile encephalopathy of obscure cause.

Infections transmitted from domestic pets to man are not frequent and are well recognized. The majority are due to fungi or helminths. Fungal infections such as *Microsporum canis* are transmitted by infected kittens to young children. Young children also ingest the eggs of *Toxocara* species from puppies and pregnant bitches. This visceral *Larva migrans* is a cause of blindness in young children.

Wounds that produce poisoning are rarely inflicted by animals. Every wound including animal bites is a potential source of infection with the *Clostridium tetani* and suitable immunization procedures are usually instituted. Bites from exotic pets such as snakes and spiders and stings from pet scorpions are rare and need no further discussion here.

Accidents and wounds about the home

It is not wise to dwell too much on the dangers in the home. We have already discussed the more obvious hazards but practically anything in the home can be dangerous particularly to children who are especially accident-prone. We shall devote the next section of this chapter to such childhood injuries in the home. First we will deal with toxic materials in the home.

Every year we learn of potential toxic hazards of more foods either due to the foods themselves or to the various additives. Toxic substances in plant and animal products have been recognized by man since the dawn of history. More or less as a result of trial and error he has weeded out the dangerous components. New foods of various sorts based on soya beans are safe so long as the toxic components are removed by heating. Crude unrefined olive oil has led to toxicity in recent years.

Poisonous plants around the home and garden have occasionally been mistaken for edible ones. The tuberous roots of monkshood (*Aconitum nepellus*) have occasionally been mistaken for horseradish. Toxicity is due to the content of aconitine which is one of the narcotic alkaloids. The leaves of the plant can easily be mistaken for those of the parsley plant.

Ill-informed collectors of field fungi may be taken unawares by some of these poisonous species that grow freely. Of these *Amanita phalloides* (the death cap) is the one most likely to prove fatal. About 30% who eat

it die from the effects of the cyclic heptapeptides and octapeptides in the fungus. The heptapeptides are the so-called phallotoxins which produce violent gastrointestinal symptoms of vomiting, diarrhoea and nausea usually about 8 h after ingestion. The octapeptides or amatoxins are 10–20 times more toxic than the heptapeptides and produce liver and kidney damage. Hepatocyte nuclei and the cells of the proximal renal tubules are specifically affected in this phase of poisoning. The principal amatoxin producing this effect is α-amanitine which works by binding to RNA-polymerase in eukaryotic cells and thus inhibiting the enzyme[25].

Hair sprays, glue, organic solvents and many other things have caused injury from time to time. Organic solvents have acquired notoriety in recent times. Many substances are used such as petrol cleaning fluids, various sorts of aerosols, fire extinguishing agents and butane. Solvents in adhesives are most commonly used and the term 'glue sniffing' has been used to encompass the activity. Solvent abuse became notable in the early 1970s mainly involving early teenage boys of any social class. It is suggested that most young abusers are merely experimenting and will not become addicts. Solvent abuse is fortunately often a group activity and isolated cases are rare. This reduces the likelihood of fatalities when the solvent is inhaled from bags over the head which may cause asphyxial death. Inhalation of solvents has social and psychiatric effects associated with euphoriant properties of the vapours. Neurological effects such as giant axonal neuropathy and cerebellar dysfunction are specific to certain compounds. For example, hexacarbons such as *n*-hexane and methylbutylketone are both metabolized to 2.5-hexanediane which causes giant axonal neuropathy[26].

There is no legal way of dealing with this problem though laws related to public order can be invoked if necessary. The general view is that invocation of the law is likely to promote rather than to restrain abuse.

A variety of other household substances may produce lung damage when inhaled. Paraquat weed killer is one of these and is intensely toxic when swallowed causing buccal and pharyngeal ulceration and diffuse interstitial pulmonary fibrosis (Figure 6.12). Polymers in hair sprays such as polyvinyl pyrrolidine can also cause damage if inhaled repeatedly but some degree of individual hypersensitivity is needed to produce effects. Diffuse interstitial fibrosis is a feature and is associated with the appearance of periodic acid Schiff-positive granules and lamellar lysosomes in pulmonary macrophages[27].

Other substances used to adorn the body can be toxic. Their effects are not always suspected particularly if they are the product of other cultures. Surma is a good example. This is a fine powder looking like mascara which has been used for medicinal and cosmetic purposes for years. It is usually applied to the conjunctiva and its name is derived from the Urdu word for antimony which was its main constituent. Shortage of anti-

mony led to its substitution by lead sulphide with consequent cases of lead poisoning particularly in Asian
children[28]. The lead may be directly absorbed from the
conjunctiva and lacrimation, eye rubbing and finger
sucking also contribute to the development of cosmetic
plumbism. Fatal lead encephalopathy is sometimes the
result. Surma is still used despite government health
warnings; education rather than legislation is likely to
be the best preventitive.

Accidents to children

About one death in every three of children between the
ages of 1 and 14 is the result of some sort of accident.
The trend has been falling since the 1960s but still in
1979 nearly 1000 children died in this way. A child
learns by exploring its home environment and all too
often parents fail to anticipate the hazards. Such things
as the overcrowded kitchen, paraffin in the lemonade
bottle, faulty window catches, loops of fabric are some
examples of the problem. The impact of a social environment is clear from the statistics. A child of social
class 5 parents is five times more likely to die before
the age of 15 than children of professional parents.

Pre-school children sustain most accidents at home
but accidents in or by motor vehicles still preponderate.
Even at 16 km/h a head-on-crash thrusts a newborn
child forward with a force of 890 N. The mother's lap
is clearly the most dangerous place for these children.
At 48 km/h the force is 2700 N. Clearly it is difficult to
hold this weight and fatal skull injury results.

After motor vehicle injuries, burns are the most frequent cause of fatal injury to preschool children. Children under five run a greater risk of dying from burns
than all other people up to the age of 65. Fires can be
caused by playing with matches but 75% of the injuries
are in fact scalds and three-quarters occur in the kitchen.
These are usually due to a child pulling receptacles of
hot water on to itself.

Less often appreciated is the danger of hot tap water.
At 60 °C it can burn through adult skin in 6 s and through
the child's skin much faster. Falls into bathtubs or
turning on the hot tap whilst in the bath are the commonest ways in which hot water injury is produced. This
is a good case for lowering standard water temperature
in hot taps to 49 °C.

Children and especially toddlers may burn themselves on stove doors and radiators or accidentally ignite
their clothing from such appliances. Sucking or biting
an electric flex can be another cause of childhood burns.

Accidental drowning in swimming pools, baths and
even buckets of water has already been mentioned.
Various foreign bodies can also lead to childhood asphyxia. Children put all sorts of things into their mouths
and since they do not develop the habit of chewing until
about 4 years of age they may choke on inadequately
masticated food of any sort. Round objects such as
balloons, peanuts and gum drops are particularly haz

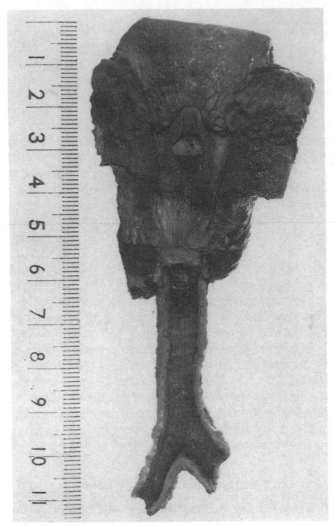

Figure 6.13   *A bolt detached from a cot blocking the laryngeal introitus of a baby found dead in its cot*

ardous because they may block the trachea entirely.
97% of objects which result in the choking of small
children are 32 mm or less in diameter (Figure 6.13).

Asphyxiation by plastic bags is a constant hazard to
children and accidental asphyxia can result in other
ways by wedging of the head between crib rails, stair
rails and ill-fitting mattresses in cots. Ill-designed cots
can provide many hazards and dangling or suspending
toys in the crib add to the danger[29]. Sturmer *et al.* have
given a concise summary of the modes of asphyxial
death involving infants and young children[30].

Children often have poor taste discrimination and
swallow insecticides, antifreeze, mothballs, petrol and
turpentine which adults would never dream of putting
into their mouths. The hazards of drugs left lying around
the home are well known. They often look like sweets.
The advent of child-proof containers for pills has helped
to reduce this hazard. Before their introduction aspirin
was the leading cause of poisoning amongst children.
Patterns of accidental poisoning of children are changing rapidly. A study in Brisbane showed 2098 poisonings
of children from 1977 to 1981. Only one child died

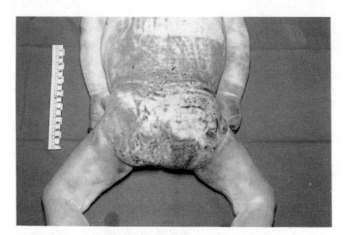

Figure 6.14 *Severe dermatitis due to repeated contamination of the skin with urine*

which is a dramatic fall in mortality. The peak incidence occurred in 1979 and has been falling since[31].

A similar pattern of decline of childhood poisoning has been reported from Newcastle[32]. Salicylates and paracetamol have ceased to be prominent causes following the introduction of child-resistant containers. The important medicines causing poisoning were found to be tricyclic antidepressants, benzodiazepines, lomotil and iron preparations. Few of the children were poisoned with household products. The number of adolescent girls admitted with self-poisoning over the period 1974–81 outnumbered the number of teenage boys admitted after ingestion of alcohol.

Unusual cases of poisoning may arise from the use of seemingly innocuous objects such as napkins and baby powder. Various chemicals applied to diapers may be readily absorbed through the buttock skin of babies. This is particularly liable in the area where the skin is often wet and macerated by ammoniacal urine. In addition, ammoniacal dermatitis increases the vascularity of the skin which also facilitates absorption of toxic substances[33] (Figure 6.14).

The hazards of marking ink were first reported at the end of the last century. This material produces methaemaglobinaemia and the child develops a slate-grey hue. Intravenous methylene blue usually deals with the condition but there have been deaths from bronchopneumonia. Dusting powders containing boric acid can also be absorbed from the skin in this way. It was used to treat napkin rashes and can lead to vomiting, diarrhoea and convulsions. The mortality is of the order of 70% in children under 1 year of age. Laundering agents such as pentachlorophenol lead to a rise in the metabolic rate. Fever, tachycardia, sweating and dyspnoea may be wrongly diagnosed as infection. Exchange transfusion will remove the phenols since most are carried in the plasma.

Baby powder which is used to dry the skin can also prove fatal if inhaled by babies in quantity. The insoluble powder enters the air passages, dries the mucosa

and immobilizes cilia. Bronchioles become obstructed and this may lead to asphyxia or subsequent pneumonia[34].

Deaths of children and injuries to children in the first few years of life occurring in the home have become a matter of serious concern to social workers and medical workers. Quite serious facial bruising, brain injury, and crushed fingers are injuries that can be caused by falls of children from 8 to 14 months of age and some have been associated with falls in appliances called baby walkers[35]. Many such injuries are, however, non-accidental and present problems in recognition and in the management of the child and its guardians.

Child abuse

Children have been subject to violence, neglect, slavery and homicide from earliest times. In the 19th century the homeless, starving child wandering in the streets was regarded as a symbol of abuse and deprivation. Home was regarded as the haven in which children could be loved and nurtured. In the 1950s it gradually became clear that the home was also a place of neglect and injury particularly for children. Caffey's description of multiple fractures in infants with chronic subdural haematomas appeared in 1946[36]. A variety of explanations was adduced to explain these injuries and they are still used in attempts to defend child abuse in the courts of law. Abnormally fragile bones due to osteogenesis imperfecta, rickets and other diseases were explanations used to explain the injuries. It was not until 1962 when Kempe *et al.* called this condition 'the battered child syndrome' that its true cause became clear[37]. Publications and discussions about the matter have increased greatly since that time. As with many medical matters better knowledge generates more cases. Nevertheless, the rate has increased in recent years and there is evidence that some cases are not reported at all.[38] Kempe *et al.*[37] said that 'many physicians find it hard to believe that such an attack could have occurred and they attempt to obliterate such suspicions from their minds, even in the face of obvious circumstantial evidence.' This is still true today and under-reporting of minor degrees of abuse is not infrequent. It is not until death occurs that the signs of earlier abuse assume their real significance.

Incidence of child abuse

The term 'battered baby' is strongly emotive and is probably best dropped in favour of maltreatment, ill-treatment or physical abuse. The definition of such abuse is also not easy because it includes all degrees of physical injury, lack of care and affection and degrees of malnutrition. Perhaps the most useful diagnostic point in these cases is the marked discrepancy in the history given by parent, foster parent or guardian and the clinical findings. Standards of child care vary in different cultures. Some still use children as slaves and soldiers and corporal punishment varies in incidence amongst different peoples. The assessment of child abuse must, therefore, take cognisance of local customs and practices[39]. In the UK the frequency of non-accidental injury to children is not accurately known. The Tunbridge Wells study group of 1973[40] estimated 4600 cases a year in the United Kingdom. Amongst these were 700 deaths and 400 children that suffered brain damage. Another study showed a rate of one per 1000 children under the age of 4 years with a death rate of 0.1 per 1000[41]. The important point is that many of the injured children remain undiagnosed and non-accidental injury remains an important cause of childhood illness with possible long-term effects of intellectual, physical and visual impairment.

The abusers

Extensive sociological, psychological and other studies have been made in order to determine those who are likely to abuse childen. Again the facts are not all clear. Child abuse is not a phenomenon of the lower social groups. It is less likely to be detected in the higher social strata because of less supervision of their children by those responsible and also because the abusers are more capable of plausible disguising of the facts relating to injury. A wide range of factors has been implicated in those who abuse their children and all do not agree on the importance of some of them. Abuse may occur at any age but the younger the child the more likely it is to be harmed and the injuries also tend to be more severe in young children.

Most of the incidents occur in the home and involve the parents or guardians though baby-sitters and other siblings have been reported as causing injuries. Amongst the adults alcoholism, sexual promiscuity, unstable marriages, cohabitation and minor criminal activities are features. These people are often immature, touchy and react quickly with poorly controlled aggressive impulses. They may themselves have been similarly abused in childhood. It is important to remember that children are also abused by the educated who are socially and financially stable. Here again there are features of free expression of aggressive impulses.

Those who abuse children have certain inherent characteristics which are difficult to change. These are aggravated by a variety of environmental factors such as poor housing, inadequate heating, shortage of food and light, lack of privacy and so on. The inherent features are often exposed when the family moves home. This is a dangerous period when the home environment is temporarily unstable and perhaps more importantly when the family leaves a well supervised environment for a new one. Medical and social records often fail to keep pace with the removal and this creates a vulnerable unsupervised period of danger to the child.

The supervisors

Supervision of families is basically the responsibility of those whose daily work brings them into contact with the children and their parents or guardians. Family doctors and those in hospital accident and emergency departments should be alert for parents showing signs of stress and who make repeated visits to surgeries or clinics with complaints about the health of their children. Many others such as paediatricians, paediatric ward sisters, community nurses and social workers are also at the forefront of detection of this important problem. Many of these children are recognized by the staff of day nurseries and nursery schools. In the UK the NSPCC, which is a voluntary organization, has taken a leading role in this field. The problem is often to get at these children and to examine them. The social worker alone, apart from the police and NSPCC, has right of access to a family in the home. Even then the baby is so well wrapped and concealed that injuries are difficult to spot. Often, however, neighbours will complain of abusive scenes and noises involving the child next door.

Despite the existence of an extensive supervisory system, together with a register of accident-prone families and health district committees to review such cases, non-accidental injury to young children persists. It is unfortunate that registers identify children that have been abused rather than parents in need of support.

Diagnosis

Early diagnosis is a challenge to all working in the field of health and welfare. This is particularly so with midwives and health visitors who spend a good deal of time observing the mother and vulnerable child in the clinic and at home. It is important to try to predict child abuse before it occurs because, at this early stage, parents are much more susceptible to help and advice than at the later stage when the pattern of abuse has been established. In this later stage fear of punishment often precludes them from seeking and accepting assistance with their problems.

Failure of maternal bonding with the child is a useful early indicator. Some of these babies are premature and have been treated in a special care baby unit[42]. Lack of early maternal contact in man and other primates can produce abnormal uncaring mothering behaviour when baby and mother are reunited. There is bound to be some deprivation of mothers with premature infants but this can be reduced by early, and frequent handling of the babies whilst they are in the incubators[43].

Lack of maternal bonding and all the other socioeconomic factors that we have mentioned set the stage for potential child abuse. The next stage is the recognition of the abuse itself. This can take many forms and often requires careful observation and thought before a conclusion can be reached.

Table 6.1 Suspect NAI especially in a child under 3 if . . .

1. Delay between accident and parents seeking help.
2. Explanation is inadequate, discrepant or too plausible.
3. The child or sibling has a history of suspicious injuries.
4. Evidence of earlier injury.
5. Child often brought to doctor or accident dept. for little apparent reason.
6. Parents show disturbed behaviour or unusual reactions to child's injuries.
7. Parents have a history of psychiatric illness.
8. Child shows neglect and failure to thrive.

Table 6.1 lists some of the indicators to be observed in the diagnosis of child abuse. Recognition of evidence of abuse is sometimes easy but is often difficult. Children may be abused in a variety of ways. This is a list of some modes of child abuse:

(1) Repeated injury
(2) Malnutrition and negligence
(3) Sudden violent fatal single injury
(4) Poisoning

In general the child may present a classical appearance of 'frozen watchfulness'[43]. He is withdrawn, unsmiling and apathetic showing no interest in people or toys. It is only after intense mothering care by hospital staff that he emerges from this frozen state. He then begins to thrive and to gain weight. This phenomenon is a useful confirmatory indicator of previously suspected abuse.

Recognition of repeated injury demands a basic knowledge of the different sorts of wounds. Not only must the wounds be recognized but thought must also be given to the possible ways in which they might have been produced. Bruises are a common feature of non-accidental injury. Different colours ranging from purple to yellow indicate that the bruises are often of different ages (Figure 6.15). A cluster of rounded bruises suggests that they may have been produced by a hand grip. It is not always easy to see bruises on a child. They are often much more evident when the subcutaneous tissues are incised at autopsy. The pathologist is often surprised by

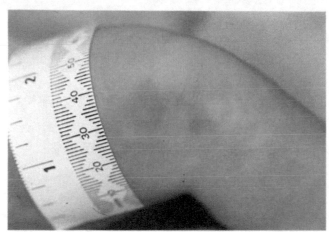

Figure 6.15   Clusters of bruises caused by hard grips with fingers

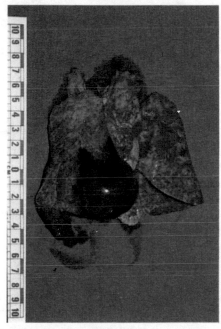

Figure 6.17   Subpleural haemorrhage over the lung due to squeezing of the chest

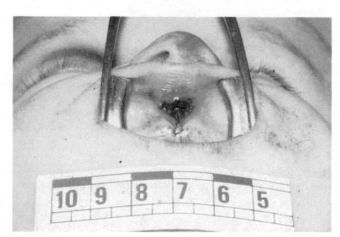

Figure 6.16   Torn frenulum of the upper lip caused by a blow across the face or by ramming a feeding bottle into the mouth

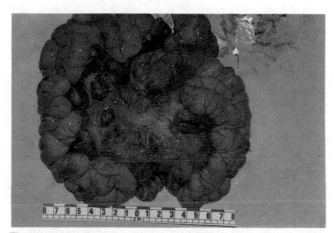

Figure 6.18   Bruising of the mesentery of the small bowel due to repeated blows on the abdomen

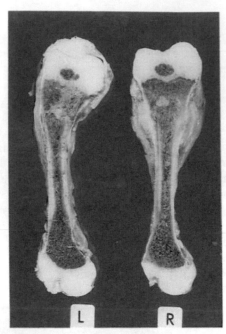

Figure 6.19 *Bilateral femoral fractures due to gripping and shaking the child, the hands of the assailant gripping the lower femora*

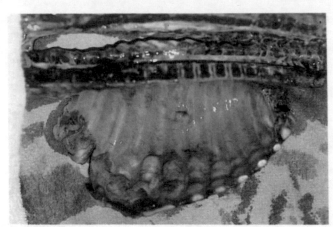

Figure 6.20 *Multiple rib fractures that have in the past been mistaken for a rickety rosary*

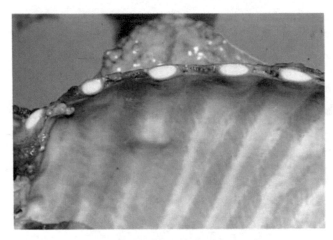

Figure 6.21 *A healing rib fracture mimicking rickets*

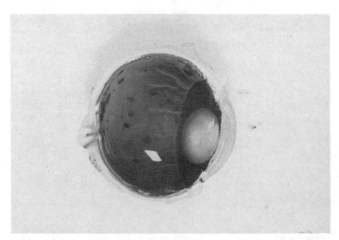

Figure 6.22 *A transected eye showing retinal haemorrhage due to either direct or indirect trauma such as squeezing the chest*

the sparse evidence of external signs of injury compared to the severity of injury to the skeleton and internal organs. Cameron[44] has provided a comprehensive account of such injuries.

The injuries may be fatal. If the child survives they form the basis of potential handicaps such as mental and visual impairment. Injuries are produced in several ways though the list is never closed. Blows produce bruises and tearing of the frenulum of the upper lip is a diagnostic feature (Figure 6.16). Internal organs such as the lung, liver and gut are also damaged (Figures 6.17, 6.18). Hand grips produce bruises and fractures of limb bones (Figure 6.19). Squeezing the child causes rib fractures at the front and back of the chest. In the past these fractures when healing have been misinterpreted as a rickety rosary (Figures 6.20, 6.21). Retinal haemorrhages may follow violent squeezing of the child's chest or neck and then form the basis for subsequent visual impairment if the child survives (Figure 6.22).

Shaking leads to organ rupture and often causes subdural haemorrhage by oscillation of the brain within the dura leading to rupture of subdural veins. Sexual abuse occurs sometimes. Cigarette burns, bath-water scalds, whipping marks and marks due to restraint with ligatures all may occur and often provide puzzling injuries that are sometimes difficult to explain (Figures 6.23–6.27).

Malnutrition and negligence are suggested by the child being underweight and often showing an extensive napkin rash. These are more difficult to interpret as child abuse and may merely be an indicator of an indigent ignorant parent (Figure 6.28).

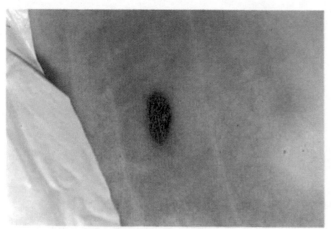

Figure 6.23 *Cigarette burn due to oblique application of a burning cigarette end. It has a characteristic 'volcanic' appearance*

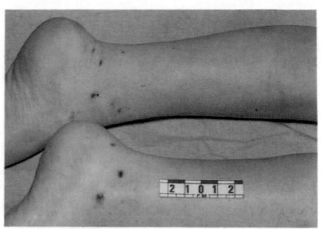

Figure 6.26 *Ligature marks around the ankles of a child*

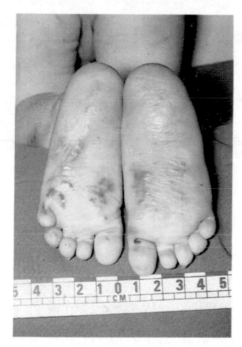

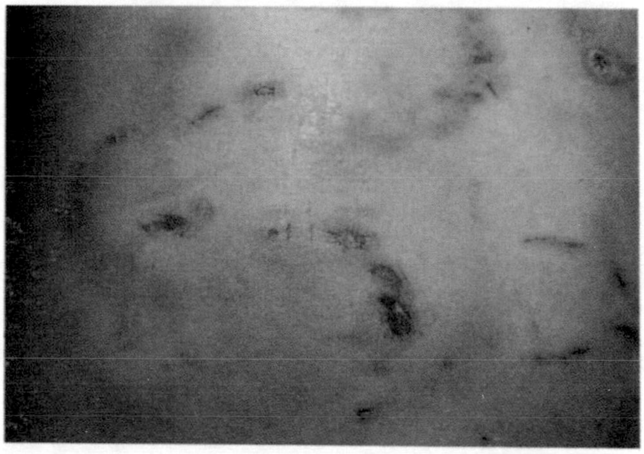

Figure 6.24 *Healed scalds on the soles of the feet*

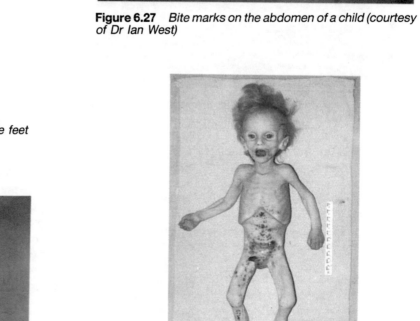

Figure 6.27 *Bite marks on the abdomen of a child (courtesy of Dr Ian West)*

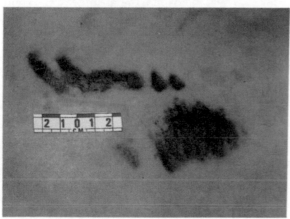

Figure 6.25 *Whip marks on the back of a child*

Figure 6.28 *Severe wasting of a neglected child. It weighed 6.4 kg at 14 months of age*

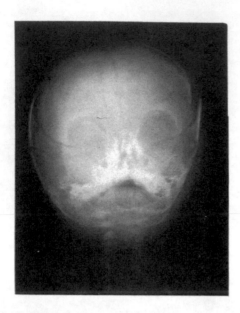

Figure 6.29 *Radiograph of fractured skull produced by banging the child's head on to a flat bench*

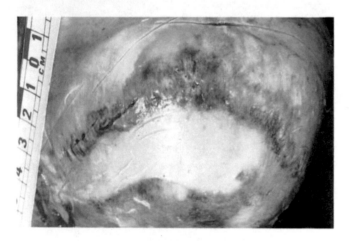

Figure 6.30 *Haemorrhage and distraction of skull sutures due to blunt injury to a child's skull*

Single fatal injuries such as skull fractures with severe brain damage may be explained plausibly by the parents. It is only when clear signs of abuse appear in a subsequent child that the possibility of abuse rather than accident is raised as a cause of death of the first child (Figures 6.29, 6.30). If one child in a family is abused there is a significant risk of other children in the family being involved later on.

Poisoning and food fads are often difficult to detect in child abuse. Several examples of poisoning of children by their parents have been reported. A variety of agents such as salt, amylobarbitone, codeine, phenformin and others were used.

Conclusions

When a doctor is called to see a child under the age of 3 years that has been injured the possibility of non

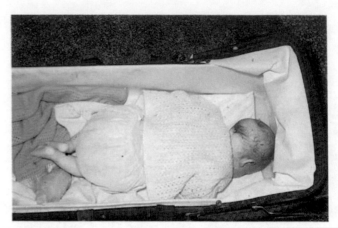

Figure 6.31 *A typical 'cot death' scene*

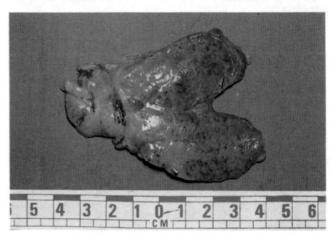

Figure 6.33 *Cuffing of bronchiole by chronic inflammatory cells from a 'cot death'. Parainfluenza virus was isolated post-mortem*

accidental injury must be considered. This has to be done carefully without any suggestion that a 'witch-hunt' is in progress.

First he has to decide if the injuries fit the explanations provided. These explanations often vary on repeated questioning. If he suspects injury he must contrive to admit the child to hospital where radiographs can be taken and colour photographs of the injuries should also be done. Whilst in hospital the attitude of the child may change and it may gain weight. These are useful diagnostic features of abuse.

If the possibility of child abuse exists the doctor must then consult widely with colleagues in the social services and other related disciplines to ensure the future care and safety of the child.

Cot deaths (crib deaths)

About 1500 young children die suddenly and unexpectedly in the home every year in the UK. They are usually only a few months old and the condition is called cot death, or crib death in the USA. A vast literature has appeared about this subject[45] but the precise cause of

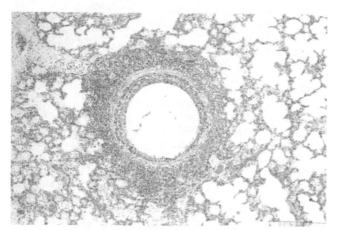

Figure 6.33 *Cuffing of bronchiole by chronic inflammatory cells from a 'cot death'. Parainfluenza virus was isolated post-mortem*

cot death remains elusive. A small number of these children are probably the victims of non-accidental injury such as poisoning with salt, aspirin and so on.

Several theories have been proposed including suffocation, viral infection, milk allergy and disorders of respiratory control. The last view is the one that has received a good deal of support based on the findings at autopsy and on studies of respiratory rhythms in near-miss cases and in the siblings of dead babies.

The usual history is of a baby aged about 3 months who may have had an upper respiratory infection recently found unexpectedly dead in its cot (Figure 6.31). Male children preponderate and they are often fed on artificial milks, often being plump, well-fed babies. Autopsy reveals very little. Petechiae are often present in the thymus, pleura and on the lungs and pericardium (Figure 6.32). These may merely represent a terminal asphyxial event. The lungs are often mildly oedematous which may again reflect hypoxia.

A number of changes have been described in various organs on histological examination and many of them suggest that the infant had suffered previous hypoxic events. Studies of the brainstem have shown astrocytic gliosis in the region of the nuclei that regulate autonomic function. Changes have been seen in the dorsal vagal nucleus and in the nucleus ambiguous. Similar lesions have been described in experimentally induced asphyxial episodes in non-human primates.

Other findings such as depletion of granules in the chemoreceptor cells of the carotid bodies, hypertrophy of the right ventricle and pulmonary arterioles also point to hypoxic episodes in these children. Abnormalities in the cardiac conducting system have also been reported indicating potential cardiac dysrhythmias as a cause of death[46]. Other workers have failed to confirm these observations.

All of these morphological findings are subject to the difficulty in finding adequate controls for comparison. Sudden infant death is the commonest cause of death

in the 3-month group of children. Apart from a few violent deaths due to road traffic or other injuries most other children dying in this age group have diseases such as leukaemia or malignant neoplasms. Such cases cannot be regarded as adequate controls for sudden infant deaths.

Apart from some disorder of respiratory control there are other theories to explain cot death. Acute viral infection has been one of them (Figure 6.33); the respiratory syncytial viruses have been particularly implicated. Anaphylactic shock due to the inhalation of cow's milk during sleep is another view that has been proposed.

At present the cause of these deaths remains obscure. The Foundation for the Study of Infant Deaths maintains active interest and research into the problem.

Bibliography

1. Jackson, R. H. and Wilkinson, A. W. (1976). Why don't we prevent childhood accidents? *Br. Med. J.*, **1**, 1258
2. Fox, R. H., MacGibbon, R., Davies, L. and Woodward, P. M. (1973). Problem of the old and the cold. *Br. Med. J.*, **1**, 21
3. Fox, R. H., Woodward, P. M., Fry, A. J., Collins, J. C. and MacDonald, J. (1971). Diagnosis of accidental hypothermia in the elderly. *Lancet*, **1**, 424
4. Besdine, R. W. (1979). Accidental hypothermia: the body's energy crisis. *Geriatrics*, **34**, 51
5. Hirvonen, J. (1976). Necropsy findings in fatal hypothermia cases. *Forensic Sci.*, **8**, 155
6. Marcinkowsky, T. and Pankowski, M. (1980). Significance of skin metallisation in the diagnosis of electrocution. *Forensic Sci. Int.*, **16**, 1
7. Wright, R. K. and Davis, J. H. (1980). The investigation of electrical deaths. A report of 220 fatalities. *J. Forensic Sci.*, **25**, 514
8. Adjutantis, G., Dritsas, C. and Iordanidis, P. (1973). An unusual occurrence of electrical burns in a case of fatal electrocution. *Forensic Sci.*, **2**, 255
9. Schwerd, W. and Schulz, E. (1978). Carboxyhaemoglobin and methaemoglobin findings in burnt bodies. *Forensic Sci. Int.*, **12**, 233
10. Perez-Guerra, F., Walsh, R. E. and Sagel, S. S. (1971). Bronchiolitis obliterans and tracheal stenosis. Late complications of inhalation burn. *J. Am. Med. Assoc.*, **218**, 1568
11. Binder, J. W. and Roberts, R. J. (1980). Carbon monoxide intoxication in children. *Clin. Toxicol.*, **16**, 287
12. Dyer, R. F. and Esch, V. H. (1976). Polyvinyl chloride toxicity in fires. Hydrogen chloride toxicity in fire fighters. *J. Am. Med. Assoc.*, **235**, 393
13. Purves, J. D. (1975). Dental identification of fire victims. *Forensic Sci.*, **6**, 217
14. Emson, H. E. (1978). Problems in the identification of burns victims. *Can. Soc. Forensic Sci. J.*, **11**, 229
15. Teige, B., Lundevall, J. and Fleischer, E. (1977). Carboxyhaemoglobin concentrations in fire victims and in cases of fatal carbon monoxide poisoning. *Z. Rechtsmed.*, **80**, 17
16. Katcher, M. L. (1981). Scald burns from hot tap water. *J. Am. Med. Assoc.*, **246**, 1219
17. Pearn, J. H. and Thompson, J. (1977). Drowning and near-drowning in the Australian Capital Territory: a five-year total population study of immersion accidents. *Med. J. Aust.*, **1**, 130

18. Scott, P. H. and Eigen, H. (1980). Immersion accidents involving pails of water in the home. *J. Paediatr.*, **96**, 282

19. Rigg, B. M. (1979). Chain-saw facial injuries. *Can. J. Surg.*, **22**, 149

20. Citron, N. D. and Wade, P. J. (1980). Penile injuries from vacuum cleaners. *Br. Med. J.*, **2**, 26

21. Dolcourt, J. L., Finch, C., Coleman, G. D., Klimas, A. J. and Milar, C. R. (1981). Hazards of lead exposure in the home for recycled automobile storage batteries. *Paediatrics*, **68**, 225

22. Ribiero, B. F. (1975). Occupation hazards in window cleaning. *Br. Med. J.*, **3**, 530

23. Maetz, H. M. (1979). Animal bites, a public health problem in Jefferson County, Alabama. *Pub. Health Rep.*, **94**, 528

24. Kearney, M. S., Dahl, L. B. and Stalsberg, H. (1982). Can a cat smother and kill a baby? *Br. Med. J.*, **285**, 777

25. Leader. (1972). Death-cap poisoning. *Lancet*, **1**, 1320

26. Leader. (1982). Solvent abuse. *Lancet*, **2**, 1139

27. Valeyre, D., Perret, G., Amouroux, J., Saumon, G., Georges, R., Pre, J. and Battesti, J-P. (1983). Diffuse interstitial pulmonary disease due to prolonged inhalation of hair spray. *Lung*, **161**, 19

28. Ali, A. R., Smales, O. R. C. and Aslam, M. (1978). Trauma and lead poisoning. *Br. Med. J.*, **2**, 915

29. Bass, M. (1977). Asphyxial crib death. *N. Engl. J. Med.*, **296**, 555

30. Sturner, W. Q., Spruill, F. G., Smith, R. A. and Lene, W. J. (1976). Accidental asphyxial deaths involving infants and young children. *J. Forensic Sci.*, **21**, 483

31. Pearn, J., Nixon, J., Ansford, A. and Corcoran, A. (1984). Accidental poisoning in childhood: five year urban population study with 15 year analysis of fatality. *Br. Med. J.*, **288**, 44

32. Lawson, G. R., Craft, A. W. and Jackson, R. H. (1983). Changing pattern of poisoning in children at Newcastle 1974–81. *Br. Med. J.*, **287**, 15

33. Leader. (1970). Deadly diapers. *Br. Med. J.*, **1**, 314

34. Motomatsu, K., Adachi, H. and Uno, T. (1979). Two infant deaths after inhaling baby powder. *Chest*, **75**, 448

35. Fazen, L. E. and Felizberto, P. I. (1982). Baby walker injuries. *Paediatrics*, **70**, 106

36. Caffey, J. (1949). Multiple fractures in the long bones of infants suffering from chronic subdural haematoma. *Am. J. Roentgenol.*, **56**, 163

37. Kempe, G. H., Silverman, F. M., Steele, B. F., Droegemuller, W. and Silber, H. K. (1962). The battered child syndrome. *J. Am. Med. Assoc.*, **181**, 17

38. McDonald, A. E. and Reece, R. M. (1979). Child abuse: problems of reporting. *Paediatr. Clin. N. Am.*, **26**, 785

39. Taylor, L. and Newberger, E. H. (1979). Child abuse in the international year of the child. *N. Engl. J. Med.*, **301**, 1205

40. Franklin, A. W. (1973). *Tunbridge Wells Study Group on Non-accidental Injury to Children.* (Spastics Society)

41. Baldwin, J. A. and Oliver, J. E. (1975). Epidemiology and family characteristics of severely abused children. *Br. J. Prevent. Soc. Med.*, **29**, 205

42. Lynch, M. A. and Roberts, J. (1977). Predicting child abuse: signs of bonding failure in the maternity hospital. *Br. Med. J.*, **1**, 624

43. Jackson, A. D. M. (1982). 'Wednesday's Children': a review of child abuse. *J. Roy. Soc. Med.*, **75**, 83

44. Cameron, J. M. (1970). The battered baby. *Br. J. Hosp. Med.*, **4**, 769

45. Kelly, D. H. and Shannon, D. C. (1982). Sudden infant death syndrome and near sudden infant death syndrome: a review of the literature 1964–1982. *Paediatr. Clin. N. Am.*, **29**, 1241

46. James, T. N. (1968). Sudden death in babies: new observations in the heart. *Am. J. Cardiol.*, **22**, 479

Chapter 7

Injury on the Road and in the Air

Patterns of injury are changing continuously as man devises new modes of transport, new firearms and other injurious devices. Seat-belt legislation has significantly reduced the mortality and morbidity from head injury to the occupants of vehicles[1]. However, the motorcycle continues to exert a constant toll of death amongst young men. The use of crash helmets has reduced injuries to the skull but serious injuries continue to occur to other parts of the body. Visceral and bony injuries lead to extensive fatal haemorrhage or to fat embolism. Fatal fat embolism can also occur following trauma to fat in the subcutaneous tissues of the unprotected limbs of motorcycle pillion passengers.

Motor and other cycle injuries

In 1960 in the UK 7000 people died and 340 000 were injured in road traffic accidents which, apart from the toll of human anguish, cost the country something of the order of 12 million pounds in medical care. Road traffic casualties are more common amongst the young (under 19) and the old (over 70) and the most frequent cause of death is injury to the skull and underlying brain. Furthermore, the motorcycle is a peculiarly lethal weapon: the fatality rate for motorcyclists is 17 times that for motorists[2]. Indeed they provide the commonest cause of death for the male under 30 years.

To take a more specific example: if we were to collect together an unrelated group of 100 000 15-year-old boys, who would just about fill a large sports stadium, we would find ourselves 1000 short in 10 years time. These would have died and 290 would have died while motorcycling. This number exceeds all the death toll, in this age group, for cancer, poliomyletis, tuberculosis,

pneumonia, bronchitis, rheumatic fever, influenza and suicide rolled together. The corresponding death toll for women would be 25. A further 17 000 of our contingent would have been injured on the roads and if all our original 100 000 had been motorcyclists the toll of death and injury would have been very much greater.

This disastrous state of affairs is not confined to Great Britain. It is found in every country where the moped, motor scooter and motorcycle are used. In 1959, for example, 1680 motorcyclists died in Britain, 2885 died in Italy, 2892 in France and 4458 in Western Germany.

The commonest cause of death for a person injured in a road traffic accident is injury to the head. This occurs in 60% of all road deaths and in 46% of deaths to those in vehicles but amongst motorcyclists it accounts for 70% of deaths. A motorcyclist is 17 times more liable to die for every mile he drives than is a motorist, a scooter rider 10 times and a moped rider 8.

Motorcycle head injury became a problem during the last war when the British Army lost two motorcyclists a day from accidents. It was in 1941 that Sir Hugh Cairns drew attention to the frequency of head injury as a cause of death in the fatal accident reports that he examined. Because of Cairns' work the wearing of crash helmets was made compulsory in the Army and Cairns showed that the helmet made of a shell of wood pulp was most effective in reducing damage to the head which was of two main kinds:

(1) Fracture
(2) Concussion followed by prolonged amnesia

Subsequently, the Road Research Laboratory looked into the design of helmets and made extensive investigations into the type of injury to the head which in turn

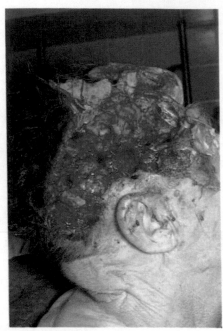

Figure 7.1 *Severe skull damage in a motorcyclist who was wearing a crash helmet but collided with a lorry at great speed*

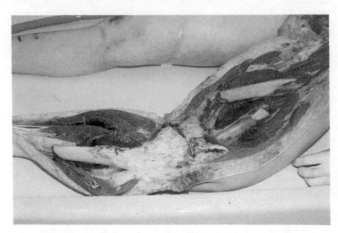

Figure 7.2 *Severe injury to the lower limbs of a cyclist following collision with a car: femur, tibia and fibula were fractured*

determines the best design for a crash helmet. The following points emerged:

(1)   Site of blow on the helmet usually corresponds to the injury of the underlying scalp and skull

(2)   More than 50% of blows are on the front

(3)   Least common on the crown

The earlier Army helmets were primarily designed to cope with blows on the crown and hence needed modification following this study. In the old helmet the internal webbing shared a blow on the crown around the skull, effectively reducing the pressure at one point. But this was of little value for blows on the side and front of the head. This was overcome by padding the shell which effectively distributes the zone of impact over a large area. A study was made of various energy-absorbing materials and the most effective was found to be cork or some synthetic substances. They have a high initial resistance to distortion followed by rapid and easy collapse. It is important to test these substances at various temperatures because on a summer day the temperature of the padding material might rise from 20 to 50 °C in 22 min if the helmet is black. If it is white the rise is to 37 °C. The highest temperature recorded was 83 °C (181 °F).

Obviously the material chosen must be capable of standing wide ranges of temperature without loss of deforming properties. Other features which were considered were the strength of the helmet itself and the degree of flexibility of the peak which should not be too soft so as to flap down over the eyes and not too hard so that the helmet rotates on the head on impact.

All the suggestions from this research were embodied in the British Standard for Protective Helmets BS 2001 and law was passed to make it an offence to sell them without the approved mark. Out of every 200 sold, three are tested, one at 120 °F, one frozen and one drenched in water. The final helmet was spaceman-type BS 1869, 1960, and studies revealed that wearing a helmet reduced risk of head injury by 33%. On roads without a speed limit it reduced the risk of death by 50%.

About 60% of riders wear helmets. The defaulters seem to be the young and the old. The reasons given are short journeys, discomfort, cost and ugliness! No helmet can save the consequence of high-speed head-on blows. A good helmet will absorb 126 J and the head 56 more. But a moving head acquires 182 J of energy at 30 km/h; a motorcyclist would do well to think before overtaking another vehicle at 100 km/h (Figure 7.1).

Of all road users, motorcyclists and pedal cyclists have much the worst casualty rates per kilometre cycled. The peak age groups are 17-19 for motorcyclists and 10-14 for pedal cyclists. The rate is 24 times that of motorists and passengers do worse than drivers of the cycles[3].

When an accident happens motorcyclists have more severe impacts than other road users. The commonest injuries are to the limbs (Figure 7.2). Of 324 patients treated for motorcycle injuries multiple fractures were frequent, the tibia being the commonest bone affected followed by the radius and ulna. Abdominal injuries were uncommon consisting of lacerated liver and spleen[4].

Laceration of the brachial plexus is one of the serious injuries peculiar to motorcyclists and though not very common the incidence is increasing. About one per 1000 seriously injured motorcyclists that survive sustain this injury. It is probably due to violent traction on the arms sustained whilst trying to maintain a hold on the motorbike on rapid deceleration. Another mode of tearing the plexus may occur on impact. The head hits

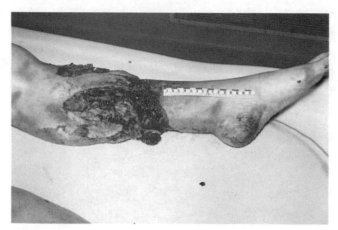

Figure 7.3 *Severe laceration of the leg of a motor cyclist involved in a collision*

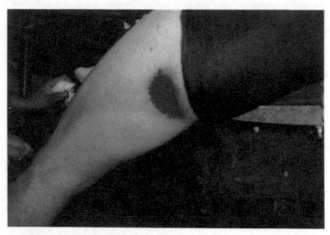

Figure 7.4 *Abrasion of the leg of a racing cyclist. The so-called 'cyclist's burn' caused by contact with the road surface*

an object and lateral flexion of the neck may tear the nerve roots on the plexus itself[5].

The motorcyclist is virtually unprotected against collision injury apart from wearing a crash helmet. Wearing heavy clothes and appropriate leg protecting boots can, however, lessen damage to the limbs. Strong footwear is essential because injuries can occur from the machine itself. This is well illustrated by injuries to the heel and lower leg that can occur when pillion riders get their feet caught in the wheel spokes when the machine is turning sharply[6] (Figure 7.3).

Pedal cycles are increasingly being used as a means of transport, partly because of the view that physical exercise helps in the prevention of coronary artery disease. There have been many changes of design over the years which enable greater speeds to be attained. Cycle racing is increasing in popularity. These races are held in various places such as open country, race tracks and within towns. Such races can involve difficult sharp corners which may cause the driver to come off his cycle at considerable speeds. As a result linear abrasions of the lateral thighs and shoulders are frequent injuries; these are often associated with puncture holes due to road surface gravel entering the skin (Figure 7.4).

In one study of pedal cycle injuries it was found that 67% suffered injuries to the head and face: of these one-fifth had skull fractures[7]. Five had subdural haematomas, four of which died. This emphasizes the importance of using some form of protective headwear. The second commonest group of injuries were fractures of the upper limbs followed by fractures to the legs. In 20% of the cases injuries were due to collision with an automobile but in only half of these was the vehicle moving. The remaining collisions were with parked cars or with cars that had stopped at junctions. All of the deaths of cyclists were due to collision with an automobile. The creation of cycle tracks goes some way towards the prevention of cycle injuries. More attention needs to be paid to suitable gear for protection of the head and limbs.

Children are especially vulnerable to bicycle injuries. There seems to be a greater risk to those using 'high-rise' machines, that is those with high handle bars and a long seat with a back rest. A number of reports have suggested that these machines are less stable than the conventional bicycle[8]. Most of the accidents occurred on borrowed machines or on those recently acquired suggesting that unfamiliarity with the cycle rather than the design of the machine itself was an important factor in causing injury.

Pedestrians head the list of road traffic injuries, children and the elderly being especially vulnerable. Britain has the highest incidence of child pedestrian casualities in Europe[9]. The rate is highest in the 5–9 age group, the risk being about 40 times greater than that of adult pedestrians. Inexperience, inattention, poor peripheral vision and poor directional hearing are all factors in children that contribute to the risk of pedestrian injuries.

The young and middle-aged adults are usually safe pedestrians unless they have been drinking. A blood alcohol of 120 mg/100 ml or more has been found to be an important factor in fatal pedestrian accidents. The elderly over 65 present the greatest problems of all. Factors similar to those in children are often operative such as inattention, poor vision and hearing.

We often speak of people being 'run over'; it would be more appropriate to say that they are 'run under'. The commonest injuries are to the legs. The pattern of injury, however, depends on the construction of the vehicle: the height of the bumper bar from the ground, the shape of the bonnet and the presence of projecting mirrors, badges and the like are all factors (Figure 7.5).

Pedestrians or bystanders may be crushed by reversing vehicles (Figure 7.6) or they may be struck a glancing blow by the side of a moving vehicle or they may be struck by the front parts of the moving vehicle. Different patterns of injury are the result (Figure 7.7).

Crushing injuries can involve any part of the body including skull, thorax, abdomen or limbs. Blows from

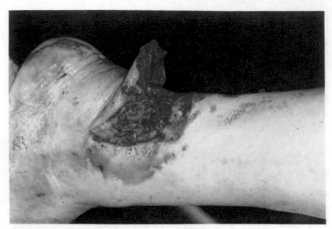

Figure 7.5   *Effects of impact of the bumper bar of a car on a pedestrian. A so-called 'run under' injury*

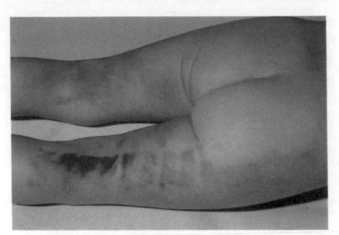

Figure 7.8   *Imprint of tyre of a vehicle on the skin of an accident victim (courtesy of Dr Ian West)*

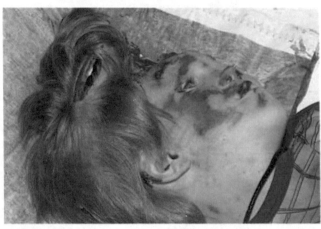

Figure 7.6   *Lateral crushing of the head by a lorry reversing into a wall*

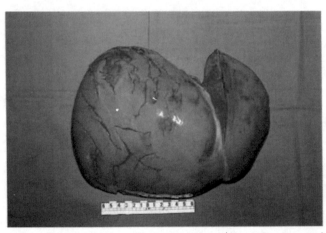

Figure 7.9   *Multiple splits in the liver surface due to crush injury*

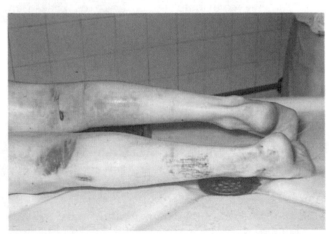

Figure 7.7   *Injury to the leg from a mudguard impact in a pedestrian*

the side of the vehicle can produce abrasions and laceration to the side of the head, limbs, chest or loins and these injuries may show a pattern which corresponds with some part of the colliding surface of the vehicle (Figure 7.8). Rib fractures and penetrating or crush injuries to lung, liver and spleen may also result (Figure 7.9).

A series of injuries may follow when a person walks in front of a moving vehicle and these depend, as we have already said, on the nature of the vehicle (lorry or car for example) and the construction of its front parts.

Primary injuries are to the legs and may occur at different levels on these lower limbs. The body may be thrown upwards on to the bonnet (Figures 7.10, 7.11) and sustain secondary injuries due to impact with the windscreen, windscreen frame or roof of the car.

Windscreen injuries can occur to people in the colliding vehicle as well as to those hit by vehicles. They are characterized by marking of shattered glass which consists of square-shaped small sections of glass derived from the splinter-proof screen. These particles may cut the skin but are often driven into it producing small

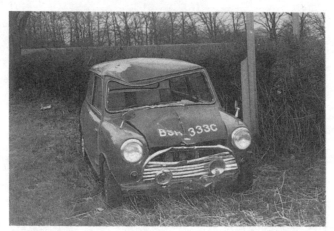

Figure 7.10   *Indentation of the front of a car by impact with a cyclist who was thrown over the vehicle*

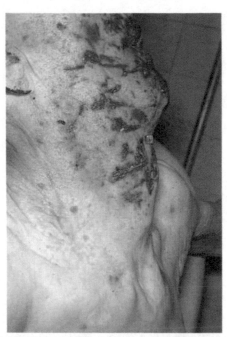

Figure 7.12   *Fragments of glass embedded in facial lacerations*

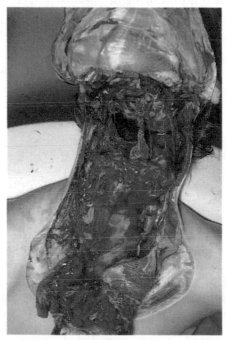

Figure 7.11   *Neck of the cyclist killed in the accident shown in Figure 7.10. Extension of the neck had caused laceration of the spinal cord and fracture distraction of the upper cervical vertebrae*

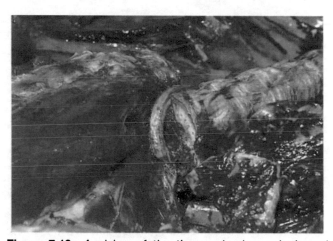

Figure 7.13   *Avulsion of the thoraco-lumbar spinal cord following a severe impact with a vehicle*

crushing injuries in which the glass fragments are embedded (Figure 7.12). The victim may subsequently pass through the windscreen and enter the car or pass over the vehicle striking the roof. The secondary injuries that result may be severe and sometimes involve hyperextension of the neck with severance of the upper spinal cord (Figure 7.13).

Further tertiary injuries may occur if the body continues its passage over the vehicle and collides with or is crushed by other vehicles following behind the collision. The patterns of injury on the corpse may therefore be multiple and difficult to interpret. The presence of paintwork in grazes and patterned tyre marks on the body may provide clues to the causation of the wounds.

The pathologist is assisted in his interpretation of such wounds by diagrams of the incident produced by the police (Figure 7.14) and photographs of the vehicles and roads (Figures 7.14–7.16). Such photographs are often taken at a later date and may not reflect accurately the conditions that existed at the time of the accident. The photographs often tend to shorten the views of the scene and the accounts of witnesses must not be accepted readily. The accident often occurs in a split second and even the trained observer may not be able to provide an accurate account. Directions of moving vehicles can often be wrong and the number of vehicles and persons involved can often be inaccurate. Any attempts to construe speeds of movement of vehicles

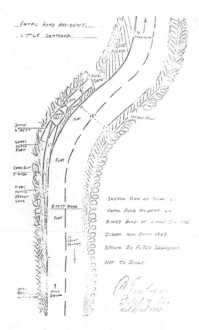

Figure 7.14   *Sketch of the scene of a road traffic accident*

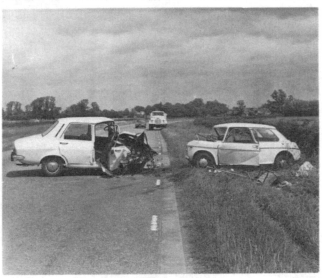

Figure 7.15   *Typical photograph of a scene of a road traffic accident*

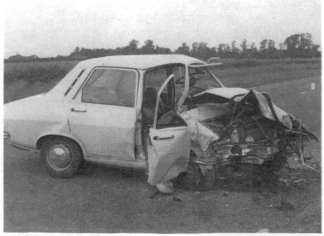

Figure 7.16   *A clear view of a vehicle involved in Figure 7.15*

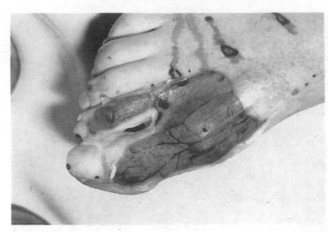

Figure 7.17   *Toe injury due to entrapment in car pedals*

and persons and force of impact should be resisted. Too many factors are often involved which prevent a reliable assessment of the situation.

Injury of occupants of motor vehicles

Occupants of vehicles also sustain injury on impact. They may suffer primary injury due to collision with parts of the vehicle itself or secondary injuries if they are thrown out of the car into the path of another or against an unresisting surface. Acceleration and deceleration injuries are common in occupants of vehicles. Violent extension or flexion of the head or the neck can break it and a variety of lacerations to internal organs can follow sudden arrest of the body at speed. These injuries have been described in Chapter 2.

Children are especially vulnerable and should never be allowed to travel on the knees of a front-seat passenger. Collision of the child's head with the inside of the vehicle can cause destruction of the skull and brain. Babies should travel in carry-cots placed transversely across the rear seats and bucket seats with belts should be provided for older children[10,11]. Amongst children the highest death rate for occupants of motor vehicles occurs in the first year of life. This is probably because they are more likely to be travelling in the front seat of the vehicle[12].

Injuries to adult occupants of cars are frequent though serious injuries have to some extent been reduced by the use of seat belts and head supports. Facial injury is the commonest type and is related to the position of the person in the vehicle. The front-seat passenger has proved to be the most vulnerable colliding with windscreen or with the dashboard[13]. Impact with the windscreen produces typical glass injury. These particles may be driven deeply into the skin and they may even be inhaled into the lungs on impact.

Additional injuries can occur to the driver of the vehicle from the steering wheel and car pedals (Figure 7.17). Stove-in chest and fractures caused by the transmission of force along the limbs are frequent.

Contrary to popular opinion rear-seat passengers are not immune from injury. In these people injury to the neck, face and thorax are common. If the impact is from the rear severe neck injuries to the lower cervical vertebrae may occur[14,15].

Not all vehicle injuries are fatal. Some may be trivial and yet prove fatal because of failure to appreciate the problem. 142 post-mortem reports of road accident deaths in the Windsor area revealed that most of the deaths were due to head and chest injuries. However, 12 died of inhalational asphyxia from nose and other facial injuries and another 18 died of blood loss due to relatively minor injuries[16]. This underlines the important role of those trying to give assistance to victims of road traffic accidents. The important things to do are to stop bleeding and maintain an airway.

Delayed injuries may also occur and are often unrecognized at the time of the accident. There are many examples of injuries to thoracic and abdominal organs. Delayed rupture of a partially torn descending thoracic aorta and traumatic thrombosis of coronary arteries are examples[17]. Tears of the left atrium and pulmonary veins if recognized early are amenable to surgical salvage[18].

A variety of intra-abdominal injuries may occur. Rupture of the diaphragm with secondary strangulation of a viscus is described[19]. Delayed rupture of the stomach is a rare event that may not present for a week or so after injury[20]. Delayed rupture of the spleen on the other hand is a not uncommon and well recognized problem characterized by shoulder tip pain. Tearing of the liver surface and pulping of the interior of the organ may also lead to delayed bleeding. Small children are especially prone because of the relatively large size of the organ. Splitting and rupture of the intestines also may follow blunt abdominal trauma in children and adults. In children the kidney is the commonest organ to be involved[21]. The kidney itself is torn or the pedicle may be torn as a result of deceleration injury.

Causes of vehicular injuries

A number of factors are responsible: the driver, the vehicle, driving conditions, road surface and so on. Vehicle factors comprise faults in design and defects that develop in use. Safety is not always the prime consideration in design: other matters such as speed, ease of driving, comfort and the like may take precedence.

So far as the driver is concerned illness contributes little to the cause of road accidents. Acute disease such as cardiac dysrhythmia and epilepsy are often difficult to assess and may be masked by severe injury. Furthermore, autopsy studies of the cardiac conducting tissues are rarely made so that a cause of sudden arrhythmias may be missed[22]. A study of 328 drivers who died as a result of vehicle accidents did not show any correlation between driver responsibility and autopsy evidence of

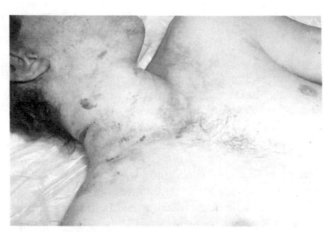

Figure 7.18 *Pattern of bruising on chest due to impression of a seat belt. The neck laceration is also caused by the belt cutting into the flesh*

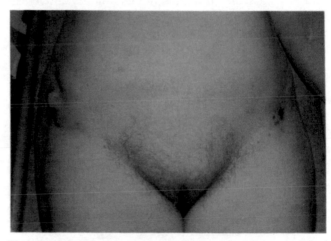

Figure 7.19 *Transverse abdominal bruising due to seat belt pressure (courtesy of Dr Ian West)*

disease and disability. Coronary artery disease was found with equal frequency in drivers at fault and those who were not to blame[23].

The dangerous effects of alcohol on the driver are well known. A sharp and immediate reduction in road accidents followed legislation in 1967 which made driving with a blood alcohol over 80 mg/100 ml illegal in the UK. Other drugs such as minor tranquillizers also impose an increased risk. Diazepam is particularly important in this respect[24].

Seat belts which may produce their own peculiar patterns of injury have nevertheless contributed greatly to a driver's safety. Belted occupants of cars are rarely killed except in accidents at high speed. A given severity of injury needs an average speed which is 19 km/h greater if the driver is wearing a seat belt. Seat belts are less effective in side crashes or when the car is crushed. Fire occurs in less than 0.5% of accidents so that fear that a seat belt might impede exit from the vehicle is no argument against belt usage[25]. Legislation in the UK was completed in 1979 making the wearing of seat belts compulsory. Road deaths declined thereafter, in particular deaths from head injury.

It is well accepted that the occupant of a car may be injured in an accident by the seat belt that is being worn (Figures 7.18, 7.19). The type of belt is important: abdominal injuries are more frequent with lap belts as compared to lap and diagonal belts[26]. Some of the injuries are due to incorrect placing and wearing of the belt such as tearing and perforation of the small bowel. Symptoms of this may be delayed for several days and surgeons should be cautious when abdominal bruising due to the belt is found in a road traffic victim.

The term 'seat-belt syndrome' was coined in 1962. A review of 3325 car occupants who were involved in accidents and who were wearing seat belts showed that some damage had been sustained in 30% but only 0.75% had serious injuries. The latter included lumbar spine, pelvic and abdominal injuries. The seat-belt syndrome includes three distinct patterns of injury which tend to be associated with abdominal injury and lower thoracic and lumbar spine trauma. Diagonal belts can produce fractures of the thoracic cage, injuries to the upper abdominal viscera and to the upper thoracic and cervical spines[27].

Abdominal injuries comprise bruising of the abdominal wall and muscle rupture. The hollow viscera may be damaged and the jejunum and ileum together with the mesentery are most often involved. There may be discrete multiple perforations of the antero-mesenteric border of the gut or the gut may be transected at points of fixation such as the duodeno-jejunal flexure or ileocaecal region. Injury to the left colon occurs next in order of frequency and then large and small bowel lesions are associated with fractures of the lumbar spine in about 28% of cases.

In addition to perforations of the bowel a condition unique to seat-belt trauma may occur. This is the so-called 'sleeve-stripping injury' in which mesocolon, serosa and muscularis are torn off leaving a mucosal tube behind. Tearing of blood vessels to the gut is a cause of bleeding and later ischaemic damage to the bowel. The mechanism of bowel injury is a combination of pressure and shear forces. As the belt tightens the compression causes sections of gut to dilate and split or burst. Flexion of the abdominal wall causes compression fractures of lumbar vertebrae and of the pelvis[28]. Dislocations without bony fracture may also occur in the same way[29].

Damage to the thoracic aorta includes dissection and rupture. The abdominal aorta is less often involved but longitudinal stretching due to pressure and flexion can lead to intimal dissection followed by medial dissection or rupture. Sometimes the separated intimal flap may prolapse into the aortic lumen and block it[30].

A variety of new syndromes associated with seat-belt injury continue to be described. Seat belts undoubtedly do present problems, for example with pregnant women travelling in cars[31] but their value in preserving life remains clear.

Mass casualties

Large numbers of casualties occur in civil strife and warfare, mass travel in aircraft and occasionally in trains and coaches and also in natural disasters such as earthquakes and the like. The patterns of injury are usually the same as the individual injuries that we have already discussed under previous headings. However, mass injuries and deaths are often associated with severe forces applied to the body and result in greater mutilation. For example, aircraft deaths are often associated with asphyxia, burning and extensive skeletal and visceral damage. Civil strife also tends to leave its peculiar label on corpses which is determined by the type of weapon used such as car bombs.

Civil strife and warfare

In recent years civil strife has dominated the scene and conventional warfare has taken a more minor role. Deaths and injury in both cases are often the result of conventional or home-made weapons and even result from deterrent weapons that are thought to be relatively harmless. Furthermore, any object such as bricks and bottles that come to hand are used as missiles. Recent events in England and in Northern Ireland have produced a spate of injuries from bricks, bottles, vehicles and truncheons used by the police in retaliation. Falls and kicks also occur in such a fracas. Sometimes the missile leaves a characteristic pattern of injury, often it does not. It is important for the surgeon or pathologist to obtain an accurate record or photograph of such wounds because they may subsequently be asked to say precisely how and by what a wound was caused.

Classification of trauma is an important part of studying the causes and effects of civil strife. This was done in Northern Ireland. The usual method of classification by external cause was found to be unsatisfactory as new modes of injury such as letter bombs arrived on the scene. The authors recommend listing of specific lesions as a more useful and practical way of classification[32]. This is the only useful way of classification of injuries when a wide range of weapons abound and new ones are continually being devised.

The so-called rubber bullet or baton was thought to be a safe deterrent. It is the descendant of the wooden club or baton and was intended to administer a blow equivalent to a hard slap. The problem is to achieve an accurate aim with it. It is about 15 cm long, 3.5 cm diameter and weighs about 140 g. It is mounted in a cannister with a charge at the base and fits loosely into a riot gun or Very pistol. It emerges from the weapon with a tumbling movement and at low velocity of about 73 m/s. If aimed at the legs it may strike the head and so on. Miller et al.[33] have reported skull fractures, lung bruising and eye injuries with this baton.

Even blank ammunition can be hazardous. Point-blank discharge of a .38 revolver will result in the

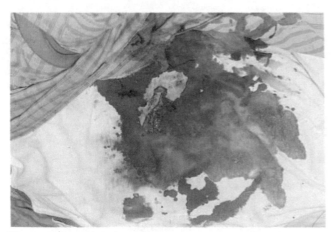

Figure 7.20 *Hole in clothing due to a gunshot discharge*

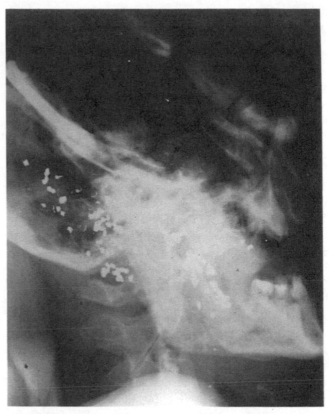

Figure 7.21 *Radiography after gunshot wounding often reveals many fragments*

powder and wadding forming a hole 6 cm deep. The adjacent tissue is also scratched. At 5 cm away from the tissue a depth of 3.5 cm penetration is still achieved. Discharge at 30 cm from the body can damage an eye and produce blindness[34].

Blast injuries received a lot of attention during the last war and were particularly studied after the detonation of nuclear weapons. In subsequent years a variety of bombs of varying power have been fabricated in the support of civil strifes. Reports continue to come in daily from all parts of the world and a large literature on such bomb injuries is now accumulating.

Letter bombs are a favoured way of creating individual injury which makes detection of the criminal difficult. The injuries occur when the letter is being opened: they tend to affect the hands, face, eyes and ears. One or more digits may be lost from the hands. The face is often lacerated and the eyeball may rupture with traumatic cataract and retinal haemorrhages. Injury to the ear consists of rupture of the drum head or damage to the cochlea[35]. Petrol bombs consist of containers holding petrol and plugged with a rag. The rag is lit before the bomb is thrown. Surprisingly they cause very few injuries[36].

Larger bombs are constructed from a range of material such as drain pipes packed with explosive and a charge of glass, nails and so on. They are detonated by fuses, tilting electrical circuit makers or by some form of chemical action. Injuries may be divided into three main groups. There is a blast effect on tympanic membranes or on the lung producing multiple haemorrhages. The latter are produced as the shock travels through the body causing parts of the lung to shear on one another with tearing of blood vessels. This is a more likely mode of injury than the suggestion that the blast wave travels down the trachea and bronchi. Flash burns and injury from flying fragments are the two other groups of bomb injury. Fragments produce a host of different effects depending upon the proximity of the individual to the bomb at the time of explosion[37]. Further injuries are secondary and are brought about by

collapse of buildings, sheets of flying glass and so on.

The use of guns in terrorist activities presents problems for the pathologist. A variety of weapons is used of different calibre and of differing power. This can make the distinction of exit and entrance holes difficult. In general, the greater the velocity of the missile the more energy it imparts to the tissues through which it passes and the greater the tissue damage. Details of wound ballistics are well described by Owen-Smith[38].

Post-mortem procedure in subjects dead of gunshot wounds differs little from other forensic practice. The important thing is to preserve evidence. Clothing should be removed with care and inspected for bullets, stains and powder marks (Figure 7.20). The clothing should be disturbed as little as possible in removal and subsequently photographed, hung up to dry and rephotographed if necessary. The position of wounds measured from the shod heel should be recorded and if possible exit and entry wounds determined. Radiography of the body is a valuable adjunct in locating missiles and fragments of metal (Figure 7.21).

Careful examination and photography of gunshot wounds is an essential part of the procedure. In doing this it is essential not to wipe away powder residues on skin, bone and other tissues. The residues can provide useful clues to the type of weapon used. In addition a study of powder residues on the hands may indicate the type of weapon fired by the individual.

Using neutron activation analysis it is possible to

distinguish different types of bullet used by their content of aluminium, copper, tin, silver and antimony. Determination of antimony levels in skull fractures has confirmed the fact that the fracture was due to a bullet rather than to some other cause. Analysis of powder residues on skin indicate that the individual fired a weapon and may point to the type of gun that had been used[39].

With contact and intermediate gunshot wounds powder is deposited on the skin and is also tattooed into the skin. At greater distances no tattooing occurs. The occurrence of tattooing also depends on the type of powder involved. For .38 calibre powder tattooing with flake powder occurs up to 60 cm. Flattened ball powder tattooes up to 90 cm whilst ball powder extends up to 1.20 m.

Aircraft deaths

Deaths from aircraft disasters present the pathologist with many problems. There are a large number of bodies to deal with, belongings to be secured, identification to be done in the face of massive mutilating injuries. Team work is essential. This is assured in the UK but in other countries, for political or other reasons, team co-operation may not always be forthcoming.

Safety measures in aircraft are not as satisfactory as they might be. Lap seat belts provide inadequate protection. Injuries to the head, chest and legs are often severe and are largely due to the cramped space with passengers situated too close to the structures in the aircraft. Fire is a common hazard and serious consideration should be given to abolishing all smoking on aircraft.

Post-mortem procedures in such incidents differ little from those in other forensic circumstances. The scale of the task, however, demands a highly organized team.

Aircraft and airports tend to produce their own patterns of illness in air passengers. Air travel is costly and the mean age of travellers is high. They are prone to vascular disease which can be aggravated by hypoxia[40]. Despite this and the development of bigger aircraft to carry more passengers, illness in the air is comparatively rare. The majority is traumatic involving burns, sprains and bruises.

Bibliography

1. Christian, M. S. (1976). Non-fatal injuries sustained by seatbelt wearers: a comparative study. *Br. Med. J.*, **2**, 1310
2. Leader. (1962). Road deaths again. *Lancet*, **2**, 709
3. Special Correspondent. (1979). Motorcycle and bicycle accidents. *Br. Med. J.*, **1**, 39
4. Deaner, R. M. and Fitchett, V. H. (1975). Motorcycle trauma. *J. Trauma*, **15**, 678
5. Andrew, T. and Wallace, W. A. (1978). Do brachial plexus injuries occur at initial impact in motor cyclists? *Br. Med. J.*, **1**, 1668

6. Ahmed, M. (1978). Motorcycle spoke injury. *Br. Med. J.*, **2**, 401
7. Guichon, D. M. P. and Myles, S. T. (1975). Bicycle injuries: one-year sample in Calgary. *J. Trauma*, **15**, 504
8. Craft, A. W., Shaw, D. A. and Cartlidge, M. E. F. (1973). Bicycle injuries in children. *Br. Med. J.*, **2**, 146
9. Special Correspondent. (1979). Pedestrian accidents. *Br. Med. J.*, **1**, 101
10. Leader. (1977). Safety of children in cars. *Br. Med. J.*, **1**, 2
11. McDonald, Q. H. (1979). Children's car seat restraints. *Paediatrics*, **64**, 848
12. Baker, S. P. (1979). Motor vehicle occupant death in young children. *Paediatrics*, **64**, 860
13. Steckler, R. M., Carras, R., Epstein, J. A. and Bazan, C. (1972). Craniofacial injuries due to impalement on an auto gearshift lever. *J. Trauma*, **12**, 161
14. Jones, A. M., Bean, S. P. and Sweeney, E. S. (1978). Injuries to cadavers resulting from experimental rear impact. *J. Forensic Sci.*, **23**, 730
15. Christian, M. S. (1975). Non-fatal injuries sustained by back seat passengers. *Br. Med. J.*, **2**, 320
16. Kamdar, B. A. and Arden, G. P. (1974). Road traffic accident fatalities (review of 142 post-mortem reports). *Postgrad. Med. J.*, **50**, 131
17. Mackintosh, A. F. and Fleming, H. A. (1981). Cardiac damage presenting late after road accidents. *Thorax*, **36**, 811
18. Noon, G. P., Boulafendis, D. and Beall, A. C. (1971). Rupture of the heart secondary to blunt trauma. *J. Trauma*, **11**, 122
19. De La Rocha, A. G., Creel, R. J., Mulligan, G. W. N. and Burns, C. M. (1982). Diaphragmatic rupture due to blunt abdominal trauma. *Surg. Gynaecol. Obstet.*, **154**, 175
20. Lloyd, R. G. (1982). Delayed rupture of stomach after blunt abdominal trauma. *Br. Med. J.*, **2**, 176
21. Seruca, H., De Bock, J. and Guttman, F. M. (1979). Renal trauma in children. *Can. J. Surg.*, **22**, 24
22. James, T. N., Pearce, W. N. and Givan, E. G. (1980). Sudden death whilst driving: role of sinus perinodal degeneration and cardiac neural degeneration and ganglionitis. *Am. J. Cardiol.*, **45**, 1095
23. Baker, S. P. and Spitz, W. U. (1970). Age effects and autopsy evidence of disease in fatally injured drivers. *J. Am. Med. Assoc.*, **214**, 1079
24. Skegg, D. C. G., Richards, S. M. and Doll, R. (1979). Minor tranquillisers and road accidents. *Br. Med. J.*, **1**, 917
25. Special Correspondent. (1978). Road accidents – seat belts and the safe car. *Br. Med. J.*, **2**, 1695
26. Hamilton, J. B. (1968). Seat belt injuries. *Br. Med. J.*, **2**, 485
27. Shennan, J. (1973). The seat belt syndrome. *Br. J. Hosp. Med.*, **10**, 199
28. Huelke, D. F. and Kaufer, H. (1975). Vertebral column injuries and seat belts. *J. Trauma*, **15**, 304
29. Smith, W. S. and Kaufer, H. (1969). Patterns and mechanisms of lumbar injuries associated with lap seat belts. *J. Bone Jt. Surg.*, **51**, 239
30. Dajee, H., Richardson, I. W. and Iype, M. O. (1979). Seat belt aorta: acute dissection and thrombosis of the abdominal aorta. *Surgery*, **85**, 263
31. Matthews, C. D. (1975). Incorrectly used seat belts associated with uterine rupture following vehicular collision. *Am. J. Obstet. Gynaecol.*, **121**, 1115
32. Rutherford, W. H. and Ferguson, D. G. (1975). The classification of trauma. Lessons learned in classifying

injuries of 1,797 patients from civil disturbances in Northern Ireland 1969–1971. *J. Trauma*, **15**, 63

33. Millar, R., Rutherford, W. H., Johnston, S. and Malhotra, V. J. (1975). Injuries caused by rubber bullets: a report on 90 patients. *Br. J. Surg.*, **62**, 480

34. Closs, J. D. (1978). Wounding effects of blank ammunition. *R. C. M. P. Gaz*, **40**, 6

35. Fawzi Abu Jamra, Halasa, A. and Salman, S. (1974). Letter bomb injuries: a report of three cases. *J. Trauma*, **14**, 275

36. Marshall, T. K. (1978). Violence and Civil Disturbance. In: Mason, J. K. (ed.), *The Pathology of Violent Injury*. (London: Edward Arnold)

37. Waterworth, T. A. and Carr, M. J. T. (1975). Report on injuries sustained by patients treated at the Birmingham Accident Hospital following the recent bomb explosions. *Br. Med. J.*, **1**, 25

38. Owen-Smith, M. S. (1981). *High Velocity Missile Wounds*. (London: Edward Arnold)

39. Ruch, R. R. and Guinn, V. P. (1964). Detection of gunpowder residues by neutron activation analysis. *Nucl. Sci. Eng.*, **20**, 381

40. Leader. (1975). Illness in the clouds. *Br. Med. J.*, **1**, 295

Index

References in *italics* are to figure numbers.

116

Printed in the United States
By Bookmasters